CHRONIC DIGESTIVE DISORDERS

ABOUT THE AUTHOR

Gaynor Greber qualified with excellence from The Institute for Optimum Nutrition in London in 1994. (Dip ION)

She was in private practice in Surrey, Kent, Sussex and Dorset for twenty-two years, specialising in gastrointestinal health. Working in a medical diagnostic clinic, osteopathic, naturopathic and physiotherapy clinics, her own established rooms and in a GP group practice.

As a Clinical Nutritionist, Gaynor combined Nutritional Therapy with the Functional Medicine approach and has improved the health of thousands of patients over the years, not only in digestive health but in those with chronic conditions and general poor health.

Gaynor holds an advanced certificate in Metabolic Nutrition, was a 'Foresight' Practitioner for Infertility and Preconceptual care, held the post of third year course Tutor at ION and was a sports Nutritionist with an International Cycling Team.

She has regularly updated over the years, attending Laboratory Test Procedures training and post graduate courses in Functional Medicine both in UK and USA.

During this time, she was, until 2021, a Senior Associate of the Royal Society of Medicine.

She is a former member of The British Association for Applied Nutrition and Nutritional Therapy. (BANT) and was registered with the Complementary Medical Association. (CMA).

She is currently a member of The Institute for Functional Medicine. (IFM)

Now, residing in Switzerland, Gaynor continues to update regularly but mainly focuses on writing books.

CHRONIC DIGESTIVE DISORDERS

Regaining Health with the
Functional Medicine Approach

GAYNOR J GREBER

Clinical Nutritionist

Paperback Edition First Published in the
United Kingdom by Alphorn Press in 2021

Disclaimer

The author does not accept liability for readers who self-medicate
without professional guidance.

Gaynor J Greber
www.gjgbionutrition.org
Cover/images from istock.com

ISBN: 978-3-9525280-5-1
Alphorn Press

In gratitude for inspiration and invaluable experience gained from all the many interesting and warm-hearted individuals that I have had the pleasure of treating over the years.

DISCLAIMER

The Treatment Plans in this book have been shown to help people with diagnosed and undiagnosed digestive complaints.

They are not intended to replace appropriate medical care but are designed to offer natural drug-free approaches to individuals who may be unaware of their full choice of treatment options.

All complex herbal or nutritional supplementation treatment should be applied under the guidance of a suitably qualified practitioner.

The author does not accept liability for readers who choose to self-medicate with the information in this book.

Contents

Foreword

Chronic digestive disorders, and indeed, digestive disorders in general, have been steadily on the increase in the human population. Often the root cause evades detection due to the vagueness or obscure symptomology presented in each individual case. Medically it is somewhat like shooting at a moving target, difficult to pin down and hard to control. In many cases, beyond those that are more medically defined, diagnosed and treated accordingly, there remains a large percentage of individuals left struggling to find any form of effective treatment for their condition. Not surprisingly, diet, lifestyle and stress can have a major role in the causation of chronic digestive disorders and therefore, they can have a significant impact on an individuals recovery when managed properly as part of a whole recovery program. Chronic digestive disorders are in all probability very much a symptom of modern day living.

Gaynor Greber has drawn on her many years of clinical experience using diet and lifestyle modification to help patients regain their health. Often, and in most cases, Gaynor has been seen as the last resort by patients struggling to find some resolve to their chronic digestive problems. Under her guidance, Gaynor has shown to have helped many difficult, long-term sufferers regain their health and return to a healthier lifestyle.

This book contains many years of clinical practice and experience condensed into each page, offering tips on self-help, but more importantly, underpins the importance of treating not only the symptoms of chronic digestive disorders, as complex and many as they can be, but also highlights the need to treat the cause.

Anyone suffering with long-standing chronic digestive disorders, especially those who may have had limited or no benefit by conventional treatments and methods, may find the answer to their health issues amongst the pages of Gaynor Greber's book.

John Stirling ND, Dip App Sc.

Testimonials

AB

I had been feeling unwell for a few years on and off with stomach cramps and bloating. Most episodes only lasted a day or so and then were resolved. However they became more frequent and I was very gradually losing weight, which was quite scary, so I decided to consult the nutritionist Gaynor Greber rather than go to a doctor for antibiotics.

Gaynor took a detailed medical history and arranged some blood and stool tests and diagnosed the parasite Blastosistis Hominis. She explained that there were natural options available to help the body's natural detoxification and immune function to eradicate the parasite, in the form of supplements and diet. I visited Gaynor every 3 months and she prescribed me a range of supplements. Gaynor gave me a special diet to follow and very gradually I got my health back. After about 18 months from starting treatment my symptoms disappeared completely and I returned to my normal weight.

I thoroughly recommend Gaynor Greber as a nutritionist.

HC

I sought the help and advice of Gaynor a while back after two years of GP visits and hospital investigations regarding my daily symptoms of stomach pains, suspected ulcer, chronic fatigue and a distended abdomen. I was given a diagnosis of IBS and referred to an NHS dietitian with a long wait. Out of frustration at this point I contacted Gaynor for advice and support.

Gaynor immediately put me on a wheat and dairy free diet with immediate relief from all my symptoms within days. Gaynor suggested that I have a hair mineral test and stool test and recommended appropriate vitamins after the results to ensure I remain in optimum health.

I personally feel that Gaynor has had a huge positive influence in my health and lifestyle. I have also cascaded my knowledge to friends and family which in turn has improved their health and lifestyles. Many of them are so impressed with Gaynor they have had individual appointments with her regarding their own unique health concerns.

I would not hesitate in recommending Gaynor to anyone who is looking to educate themselves towards a more positive and healthy lifestyle.

CWS

Gaynor has radically changed my life for the better.

Without her incredible guidance and intellect, I would be in a very different place.

I don't know if I will ever have the luck to find anyone as well-informed, widely-read and analytical as Gaynor, so I count my blessings that I found her and was able to work with her.

I hope that this book can help other people in the same way that Gaynor helped me.

CB

I originally came to Gaynor for help in 2011, because I was suffering greatly with problems in my digestive system. This ranged from having a lot of wind and discomfort on a daily basis, to over a period of a few months having several episodes of severe nausea, pain, diarrhoea and being sick. Gaynor had me take a stool test which was very revealing, showing I had parasites, bad bacteria, candida and a host of other nasties in my gut. Gaynor put me on a strict diet for 3 months while prescribing a number of natural supplements, all designed to deal with the issues. I more or less immediately started feeling better and by the end of the 12 weeks was back to my normal happy self. I felt great!

Then in 2017/2018 I started having problems again, having become less attentive to my diet. I went to see my GP as well as getting back in touch with Gaynor. My GP was very kind and blood tests revealed I did not have any serious illnesses, but he basically said that it was IBS and there was nothing he could do. Gratefully Gaynor did not say the same! We did another stool test and I am doing another 3 month programme adhering to a diet and taking supplements. I again am feeling really well even while on the diet and supplements, and I know I will be back to perfect gut health once we are all done.

If you have any issues with your digestive system, I would like to encourage you greatly to get in touch with Gaynor. Her knowledge, expertise, and experience where it relates to digestive health are second to none. I will always be very thankful for her help and I highly recommend her!

PC

I had been suffering from a skin condition (seborrhoeic dermatitis) for some time and the problem was not improving despite frequent consultations with my GP who prescribed a range of medication including cortisone cream. Nothing seemed to work and due to the nature of the medication it was only suitable for short-term use. As soon as I stopped applying the medication the condition flared up again.

I approached Gaynor as I knew she was a highly qualified practitioner in, and a great advocate for, nutritional therapies.

Gaynor has a wealth of knowledge and experience in this field and prescribed for me a diet plan and identified the necessary supplements to rebalance my biochemistry. The positive effects are clearly evident and the symptoms are all but totally cleared. I'm confident that after a further short period of time Gaynor's programme will have completely cleared up my skin problems.

Other, more unexpected benefits from following Gaynor's recommendations have been a total absence of indigestion symptoms and also an absence of headaches, which I now realise must have been connected with my diet.

Introduction

Having spent over twenty-two years in clinical practice, treating numerous patients with digestive disorders, I have recognised that a great need exists for a comprehensive reference guide, to help people navigate through the complex and often confusing array of symptoms associated with digestive complaints.

Pain, illness and debilitating health issues are hard to deal with when not directly linked to lifestyle and diet but consider the plight of individuals who suffer with chronic digestive disorders, who struggle on a continual daily basis, with the stress and strain of fluctuating symptoms – that are liable to alter and change form with any given food or fluid intake.

There are many excellent books written on improving digestive function, but digestive disorders do not come neatly packaged with a given set of symptoms and a clear view of how to treat them. Symptoms can be extremely varied, highly individual and prey to numerous different factors – genetic make-up, biochemical individuality, levels of stress, body toxic load, diet and lifestyle considerations and digestive adequacy.

My personal professional experience gathered over many years – specialising in digestive disorders, has provided me with a clear insight into what works well clinically; when a fully comprehensive assessment is undertaken to investigate links between presenting symptoms and biochemical imbalance – nutrient deficiencies and dietary/lifestyle trends. Personal individual treatment plans are designed accordingly, depending on the biochemical analysis using only holistic non-toxic drug-free therapy. Successful outcomes over the years are in my eyes, an indication that Nutritional Therapy based on the Functional Medicine approach offer readers trusted, clinically proven, well founded natural healthcare options that deal with the root cause of ill health at a cellular level.

Each practitioner works according to his own professional instincts, experience and philosophy. You, the reader knows your body best and gathering knowledge to make informed decisions, can positively turn your health around. It is not in your best interest to be a passive participant in the quest to heal your body. The generic orthodox medical approach for digestive disorders is geared towards medication for symptom management only. The underlying cause of the health problem is not generally a matter of concern, therefore a return to good health is unlikely.

Being treated as an individual with appropriate, specifically designed treatment plans for your personal body make-up and metabolism, will enable your body to reverse, repair, restore and heal, allowing you to regain a state of optimum renewed health. In order that you can achieve digestive wellness, you first need to achieve robust health from within. The beginning part of this book aims to provide you with the information and background on why and how chronic digestive disorders can develop. By understanding the underlying root cause of your digestive health condition, you will be in a better position to initiate an action plan and start making positive efforts to help yourself on the road to better health. In later chapters I provide comprehensive treatment plans for all common digestive disorders, this is in the form of both self-help advice, easy to understand and to put in practice or for complex nutritional and herbal treatment – with the help and advice of a qualified Nutritional or Functional Medicine practitioner.

Armed with knowledge in this book about the astonishing workings of the human body you can hopefully – with confidence – follow these guidelines and learn how to conquer your digestive health problems for once and for all.

If you understand why you suffer from certain symptoms – the background behind the development of digestive complaints, and why a certain action is necessary to get better, then you are fortified with enough information to take away the fear, distress and suffering. The forceful positive power of your mind will see you through and provide support for emotional and mental strength that plays an important role in the process of healing.

The human body is never static, it is constantly evolving and changing; once you recognise the vital part you can play in providing the necessary nutrients the body requires in order for all the body systems to function optimally, then this alone is the key to reversing your symptoms and for you to look forward to a life of good health and well-being.

CHAPTER ONE

Gastrointestinal Health

'All disease begins in the gut'
Hippocrates 460 BC

Digestive health problems – are one of the most common reasons for seeking medical help.

A recent study of 2,000 British adults showed that 86% have suffered some form of gastrointestinal problems over the last year. Amazingly 30% blamed stress as the main cause of their symptoms, but only 26% of participants considered poor diet as a contributory factor.[1] This is a shocking indication that diet in general appears to rank low on the list of priorities in people's minds: dietary changes to a healthy dietary balance that is so vital for keeping the gut in good condition and functioning well is not generally on the list of options.

20% of the UK population suffer with IBS – Irritable Bowel Syndrome.

The prevalence is thought to be higher than this as many people with the disorder do not seek medical help. People with a long history of IBS are less likely to improve and more than 50% of sufferers will continue to have symptoms after 7 years.[2]

A study in 2015 stated that over 1 million residents in the USA and 2.5 million in Europe are estimated to have IBD (Inflammatory Bowel Disease).[3]

Throughout the developed world there appears to be an alarming world-wide epidemic in digestive health disorders, interestingly the figures are highest in Europe and northern USA, the countries where the highest level of processed food exists. The lowest incidence of gastric complaints come from underdeveloped countries where indigenous unprocessed foods are eaten.

The message is quite clear in these studies – for the benefit of your health, and to avoid developing digestive health problems, the diet needs to be well balanced, wholesome, unprocessed and nutritionally rich. Fresh produce should be the focus – that will nourish the gut and keep you in sound digestive health. Making a determined effort to try to avoid all the thousands of damaging chemicals that are put in food today will be a huge step in helping you reverse the symptoms of poor health. This disastrous world-wide trend in unhealthy eating patterns and rising digestive health problems could be totally avoided if more awareness was made on what damaging chemicals people are ingesting with their food.

Healthy dietary balance is the main consideration in keeping the gut in a heathy state. As you read through the book, you can gather vital information that indicates the correct conditions required for healthy gut function: the negative influence of faulty food choice, what types of food to avoid, how to achieve a healthy lifestyle and many other factors which influence the development of digestive disorders. Most importantly you can learn what action you can take to correct and reverse poor digestive health.

Toxins interfere with efficient functioning of all body systems and displace vital nutrients.

The more toxic and stressed the body becomes from intake of food additives, pesticide and herbicide residues in the food supply, the harder it needs to work – to digest food, absorb nutrients and produce energy. The body will struggle to detoxify toxins, metabolise and excrete this waste material, especially if existing on a poorly balanced nutrient deficient diet, and suffers from inadequate rest and sleep. Healthy metabolism is also compromised by negative effects from regular stimulant intake in the form of sugar, coffee and alcohol. Repetitive bad habits – over time – can be a recipe for disaster.

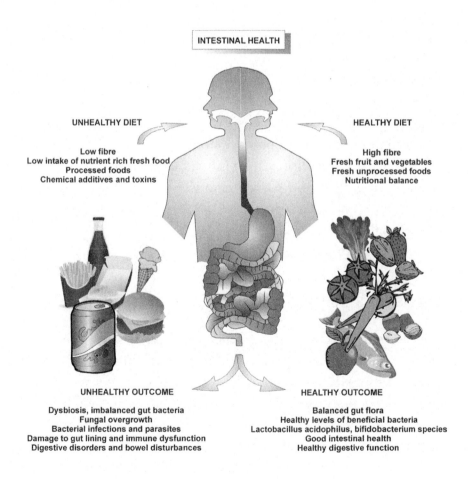

INTESTINAL HEALTH

UNHEALTHY DIET

Low fibre
Low intake of nutrient rich fresh food
Processed foods
Chemical additives and toxins

HEALTHY DIET

High fibre
Fresh fruit and vegetables
Fresh unprocessed foods
Nutritional balance

UNHEALTHY OUTCOME

Dysbiosis, imbalanced gut bacteria
Fungal overgrowth
Bacterial infections and parasites
Damage to gut lining and immune dysfunction
Digestive disorders and bowel disturbances

HEALTHY OUTCOME

Balanced gut flora
Healthy levels of beneficial bacteria
Lactobacillus acidophilus, bifidobacterium species
Good intestinal health
Healthy digestive function

HOW HEALTHY IS YOUR INTESTINAL TRACT – ARE YOU ONE OF THESE DESPERATE PEOPLE NEEDING URGENT ADVICE?

Do you suffer with:

- Irritable Bowel Syndrome, IBS is a 'blanket term' given by medics for a series of symptoms with no identifiable pathology
- Food sensitivities or intolerance
- Allergies
- Bloating, flatulence, griping gut pains
- Heartburn, indigestion
- Headaches
- Aching limbs
- Fatigue
- Constipation, diarrhoea or loose stools
- Inflammatory skin disorders or inflammatory disease
- Colitis, ulcerative colitis, diverticulitis
- Crohn's or Coeliac disease
- Duodenal or gastric ulcers
- Gastritis, hiatus hernia

DISTRESSING SYMPTOMS TO DEAL WITH

If you are suffering with any chronic digestive health problem, it is well recognised that they are the most confusing to understand and deal with. Many symptoms indicate that all is not well in the digestive tract, however taken collectively the focus should be on correcting any suspicion of faulty diet or lifestyle, any regular trends that you may feel *stress* your body.

As you start to suffer with digestive health symptoms, it is very difficult for a lay person to navigate through the myriad pathways of imbalanced biochemistry, which can result from or contribute to digestive disorders. Once you have left the doctor's surgery – having been told perhaps that your test results are negative – there is no disease present and critically that there is little to be done: you are then left with few options – except learn to live with the symptoms, try popular *fad* dietary approaches or perhaps take antacids or other drugs to relieve the symptoms.

You are left baffled by the advice, struggle to deal with a future of dietary restrictions or perpetual experimentation with different food options in the hope that your very sensitive digestive system will settle down and you will no longer have to eat with fear and worry that your stomach and bowels will react in a distressing way to what's on offer on the dinner plate.

You do not fully understand what foods upset you, which combinations are good or bad, the whole eating process is dominated by fear, worry and tension. Meanwhile you continue to suffer almost daily or whenever you eat certain food combinations or items of food that you consider 'safe'.

The picture becomes more confusing as you fail to work out why you react differently to certain food categories that you may have tolerated a while before. New pictures of intolerance may emerge, or a food sensitivity may suddenly clear when the food is presented in a different form, either cooked or uncooked or eaten at a different time of day. These symptoms are extremely distressing to live and deal with in a busy modern lifestyle. Stress has a direct negative effect on digestion, so it can contribute to your symptoms when you are in a constant state of worry or turmoil. When digestion is not working well, other signs of poor health can develop in the body.

YOUR GUT FEELING

You may be feeling under par and suffer with a range of symptoms, such as headaches, poor skin quality, lack of energy, insomnia, hormonal imbalance or frequent infections that you feel are unrelated to the gut.

In fact, body systems are holistically – intrinsically linked and faulty digestion can cause toxic bowel syndrome where undigested fermenting toxic matter that accumulates in the gut, not only favours harmful microbial overgrowth but can get re-absorbed back into the blood stream.

The health and integrity of the intestinal lining is totally dependent on optimal function of the body defence mechanisms; the tight junctions in the lining that prevent undigested matter and toxins from migrating into the blood stream. With an unhealthy diet and a disturbed microbiome – *the total mass of micro-organisms in the gut* – the intestinal mucus membrane that lines the tract can become more permeable. The tight junctions between the villi – the little projections on the lining wall can develop gaps that allow undigested food particles, toxins and unhealthy microbes to enter the bloodstream.

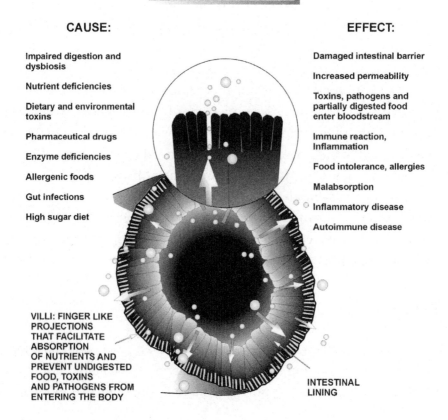

LEAKY GUT SYNDROME

CAUSE:

Impaired digestion and dysbiosis

Nutrient deficiencies

Dietary and environmental toxins

Pharmaceutical drugs

Enzyme deficiencies

Allergenic foods

Gut infections

High sugar diet

EFFECT:

Damaged intestinal barrier

Increased permeability

Toxins, pathogens and partially digested food enter bloodstream

Immune reaction, Inflammation

Food intolerance, allergies

Malabsorption

Inflammatory disease

Autoimmune disease

VILLI: FINGER LIKE PROJECTIONS THAT FACILITATE ABSORPTION OF NUTRIENTS AND PREVENT UNDIGESTED FOOD, TOXINS AND PATHOGENS FROM ENTERING THE BODY

INTESTINAL LINING

This situation is described as *'leaky gut syndrome'*. As these toxins pass through the tight junctions, they can initiate an immune response as a huge proportion of your immune cells live within the gut, and this can lead to any number of health problems developing. When a person is chronically constipated the waste material from food can cause toxic bowel syndrome which damages the gut lining and ultimately causes toxic substances to be re-absorbed into the bloodstream. If the lining becomes compromised and challenged by any of these scenarios, and an immune response is triggered – this can lead to food intolerance, onset of inflammatory processes in any part of the body and in some cases the development of auto-immune disease.

HEALTHY BOWELS – THREE MEALS IN – THREE MEALS OUT

Bowels can contain:

- By-products from partially digested food
- Bacterial matter that is fermented and putrefactive
- Undigested protein material which promote immune reactions and inflammation
- Pathogenic material from chemical food additives, toxins and wastes

For maintaining good health, stools which should not be compacted and hard should pass within 12 to 24 hours, this is called the *transit time* which is the time it takes for food to pass through your intestinal tract. It is variable and can take much longer depending on many factors: stress levels, fibre and water content in the bowels, fatty acid content and composition of the faecal matter. Calcium and magnesium – the minerals which regulate muscular contraction and relaxation to aid *peristalsis;* the movement necessary to help the material along the intestinal tract, also need to be present in the diet and in the correct balance.

Ideally, one day's meals should have been digested and the waste material excreted before the next day's meals come along.

NUTRIENTS REQUIRED FOR DIGESTING FOOD

CARBOHYDRATE	Magnesium, manganese and vitamins B1, B2, B3 and B5 are required to metabolise carbohydrate in your diet, to break down the glucose produced from these foods, in metabolic conversion stages, before the final conversion into energy which takes place in the cell, in what is known as the Krebs cycle. Vitamin C, CoQ10, iron and copper are also required with the B vitamins in this final process of energy production
FAT	Magnesium together with biotin and vitamins B1, B2 and B5 are required to metabolise fat in your diet. Following the initial breakdown into fatty acids, metabolic enzyme action works in stages for further conversion in the Krebs cycle in the cell
PROTEIN	Zinc, magnesium, folic acid and vitamins B2, B6, and B12 are required to metabolise protein in your diet. Following this process, it passes by enzyme action into the Krebs cycle in the cell

YOUR INTESTINAL TRACT –
THE CORNERSTONE OF GOOD HEALTH

Intestinal health is critical to the overall health of the human body, it is the very foundation for healthy function of all body systems.

Digestion cannot function well without a varied healthy diet containing all the nutrients mentioned above. Illness will develop if food cannot be broken down adequately. There are dozens of other vital nutrients we require in our daily diet to give us energy, and re-build cells. It is not only calories but the nutrients within the calories that our bodies require.

THE GUT

Influences health of all body organs and regulates efficient function of all body systems.

Gut health is established in the first days of life, by the diversity of an infant's micro-flora; the colonies of various microbes that live in the gut and throughout the body.[4] At birth the intestinal tract is sterile but quickly becomes colonised by a multitude of microorganisms through the journey through the birth canal into a world teeming with microbes. Breast milk helps the baby establish levels of healthy bacteria and contains antibodies to help protect against infection. Medications and antibiotics taken throughout life, can disturb this fine balance and alter or impair the rich healthy colonies of good bacteria and cause systemic ill health.

Healthy micro-flora in later life provide a valuable defence against infection and disease and will play a major part in determining your state of health, potentially influencing the course and development of disease throughout life.

LIVING IN HARMONY WITH BUGS IN YOUR BODY

The teeming diverse assortment of micro-flora associated with the human intestinal tract, is called the *microbiota*. It contains varied colonies of over 100 trillion microorganisms, including healthy and non-healthy bacteria, viruses and fungi, that help control amongst other vital functions – digestive and detoxification processes.

These body bugs have an approximate weight of between 4–5 lbs and far outnumber body cells by 10 to 1, they reside not only in large numbers in your gut but throughout your body. The gut microbiota colonies reside in a symbiotic fashion within us – the host – as an advantageous association of two different organisms living attached to one another.[5]

They thrive within the warm, dark and moist intestinal area and you provide the raw materials for their existence and survival from your diet – the correct type of fibre, nutrient rich, well balanced food that promote colonisation in the gut of the two most important species of healthy bacteria such as the Lactobacillus found in the small intestinal area and the Bifidobacterium found mainly in the large bowel. Their health depends on you and your health depends on them. Microbial colonisation is influenced by gastric acidity, the transit time of food passing through the gut, the quality of your diet, peristalsis movement, and any exposure to microbial infection.

These micro-organisms influence the immune response and inflammatory processes; approximately 70% of the immune cells reside in the intestinal lining, and it has been estimated that nerve cells in the digestive system outweigh the number of nerve cells in the spine. You can well imagine the effects on your digestion from feeling 'butterflies in the stomach' or having a nervous tummy. Digestive processes switch off under stress, this is a prehistoric survival mechanism, so you can picture how important it is that you maintain a healthy gut environment of beneficial healthy bacteria and do all you can to avoid unnecessary stress.

The microbes can 'talk' or signal chemically to one another and send signs throughout the body to influence other body systems. They can influence the way your inherited genes are expressed in terms of health and disease, define how well your body functions, within all the interconnected biochemical systems.

The microbiota determines how well we utilise our diet and our ability to digest well, detoxify damaging toxins, balance hormones, handle stress, control resistance to disease and infection, maintain mental clarity and concentration, enjoy good energy levels, and to preserve a healthy brain function. The beneficial bacterial species work hard to keep the body healthy, controlling how we feel and behave, what mood we are in, and in fact all our brain activity.

However, all these beneficial effects – if gained – can be quickly lost if disease-causing microbes multiply into an unhealthy overgrowth. The main cause is poor dietary choice causing imbalance in the diversity of healthy bacteria in your microbiota and nutrient deficiencies. Stress, lack of rest and living life in the fast lane can exacerbate this and quickly lead to digestive disturbances and ill health. You can live healthily when these non-beneficial organisms are kept under control by healthy species as they exist naturally in our body – but if they start to multiply in response to an overload of stresses and toxins, the microbiota becomes compromised and that can be an underlying cause of ill health.

The colonies of various organisms are unique to your body and are influenced by your diet, lifestyle, medication and toxin exposure.[6] Most of the bacteria in the gut should be of beneficial species, however, under unfavourable conditions mentioned above, things can start to go badly wrong with non-beneficial microbes starting to proliferate, causing yeast, fungal or bacterial overgrowth. This sets the scene for possible opportunistic parasitic infections.

At this point you would most definitely be feeling the effects of all this disruption in your gut and digestive dysfunction starts to become a problem. The first sign of trouble may include bloating, flatulence from undigested matter in the gut that starts to ferment and produce gases, which can proceed to griping pains, loose stools, food sensitivities and food intolerance.

Assessing the gut environment with comprehensive digestive stool analysis gives a practitioner an enormous amount of information about the state of your gut, the diversity of beneficial microbes, whether there is any overgrowth of undesirable micro-organisms and whether your digestive system is functioning well. This includes digestive enzymes and stomach acid assessment, level of fibre, your acid alkaline balance, fatty acid distribution and whether inflammatory markers are present.

Once any imbalances are dealt with and rectified, the gut can heal itself, which it does very successfully with inbuilt systems of repair, given the right conditions and nutrients.

Treating these symptoms with medication does not address the underlying root cause of the health problem, so nothing can improve, in fact to the contrary, symptoms may increase in severity. Side effects of medication for chronic digestive disorders only make matters worse by upsetting healthy bacterial balance, damaging the gut lining and interfering with finely-tuned digestive processes. Dependence on antibiotics for gut infections, harms and destroys not only the bad bugs in your very sensitive intestinal flora but also the healthy beneficial bacteria.

A 2013 study suggests that a potential therapeutic treatment for gut disease could be achieved by supporting the microbiome with beneficial bacteria.[7]

This approach far outweighs – in terms of health benefit, any form of medication. By replacing healthy species of bacteria that support eradication of disease causing microbes, intestinal health is preserved. The body can work in tune with nature and no damage occurs in the healing process.

By consuming healthy raw local foods, rich in natural enzymes as

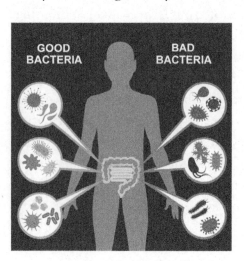

opposed to 'dead' foods that have had their enzyme life-giving vitality stripped from them by supermarket chilling procedures – you can improve your digestion and gut flora. Healthy pre-biotic foods contain vegetable fibre that healthy bacteria thrive on. There is more on this subject in chapter 6.

CHAPTER TWO

The Cause and Effect
of Chronic Digestive Disorders

*'The secret of change is to focus all your energy,
not on fighting the old but in building the new.'*
Socrates 469 BC

One third of UK GPs surveyed, commissioned by CORE said they felt inadequately equipped managing non-red flag gut symptoms, 17% found treatment of IBS most difficult. They expressed the opinion that more information on diet and lifestyle was required, especially for minor complaints such as bloating and flatulence and drew attention to a fundamental issue facing digestive disorder management in UK – people's potential to determine when it's appropriate to see a doctor.[1]

One of the most common complaints that I came across whilst in practice, was that GPs couldn't offer any supportive advice on diet and lifestyle once they had found there was no diagnosable digestive disease to deal with. Thousands of people continue to suffer gastric complaints without having the knowledge of how to manage and control their symptoms. By understanding the limitations of doctors to deal with chronic digestive symptoms, you should consider the necessity of taking health in your own hands and see what you can achieve with self-help advice. This book is intended to provide you with guidance to follow a pathway to improved health.

GPs are under enormous daily pressure, dealing with emergencies and acute sickness; dealing with chronic digestive health disorders, without evidence of a disease to treat, is time consuming and unlikely to produce positive results. It seems more prudent to refer on to experts in the field. I have had numerous referrals from GPs over many years in practice. This can relieve pressure within the National Health Service.

WHAT CAUSES DIGESTIVE DISORDERS?

- Sugar, alcohol, dietary stimulants, processed refined food
- Unhealthy eating habits, imbalanced meals, inadequate chewing and rushed meals
- Altered body pH – acid/alkaline imbalance from highly refined carbohydrates
- Deficient or excessive stomach acid, low production of digestive enzymes
- Nutritional deficiencies from a poorly balanced diet
- Excessive stress levels
- Microbial imbalance in the gut – bacterial, fungal or parasitic infection
- Toxic bowel and poor detoxifying processes
- Constipation and dehydration, lack of movement and exercise
- Low dietary fibre intake
- Medications, drugs and synthetic hormone treatment

'If a person wishes for good health, one must first ask oneself if he is ready to do away with the reasons for his illness, only then is it possible to help him.'
Hippocrates 460 BC

LIFESTYLE FACTORS – EFFECTS ON DIGESTIVE HEALTH

ALCOHOL – hampers the action of normal reflexes and slows down physical and mental activity which reduces reaction time in thought processes. If acid-promoting alcohol is taken on a regular basis, it disturbs the acid alkaline balance in the gut which can hinder the production of digestive enzymes. Alcohol also affects metabolism of many nutrients and reduces uptake of B vitamins, zinc, vitamin C and magnesium from the diet. Zinc and vitamin B6 are needed for producing stomach acid, so protein digestion may be affected. As far as the body is concerned, alcohol acts as a poison and as valuable nutrients are used up to help detoxify ethyl alcohol, the nutrient content does not contribute to any replenishment.

Red wine contains pigments that have been shown to have antioxidant properties, but it is far better to obtain these from the fruits themselves instead of putting added strain on the liver to detoxify the alcohol effect.

Alcohol and yeast promotes fungal overgrowth in the human body and can place extra strain on our digestive function. Being high in calories, with no nutritional value, a healthy body can metabolise occasional alcohol in moderation, but any sufferer with digestive problems should seriously avoid alcoholic intake.

Our digestive health depends on a slightly alkaline pH of the body, if acidic tendencies arise through diet or stress, digestive function which is very finely tuned to the (acid/alkaline) level of the body can become compromised.

SMOKING – has an extremely negative effect in the human body, one puff of cigarette smoke contains between 1200–4000 different chemicals.[2] Cigarette smoke contains about twenty poisonous gases, and thirty cancer causing agents, even radioactivity is introduced into cigarettes through fertilizers sprayed on the tobacco leaves. The paper that rolls around the tobacco is soaked in a carcinogenic liquid that encourages slow burning. The higher the toxins taken into the body, the more strain on the digestive and detoxification systems. Valuable nutrients are also used up in liver detoxification processes that must metabolise the chemicals inhaled with smoking.

PRESCRIPTION DRUGS – can deplete your nutritional status, many brands of drugs can affect your levels of B vitamins, zinc, calcium, magnesium, Vitamin C, potassium, iron, selenium, sodium and coenzyme Q10. It is well recognised that drugs have a negative effect on your gut flora – the very precious invaluable microbiota. Drugs also need metabolising down liver detoxification pathways which need nutrients to function.

COFFEE – acts as a stimulant on the central Nervous System, coffee beans contain both theobromine and theophylline, chemicals which also have the same stimulatory effect as caffeine. Dietary stimulants can cause adrenal stress by constantly activating the natural stress response – 'the feel-good effect' – resulting in an adrenalin rush, which activates hormones to raise blood sugar levels in the blood. A few hours later this is followed by a dip in blood sugar level with the pattern repeating itself, this is where addiction can take a hold.

The result of regular coffee intake is constant stress on the endocrine (hormonal) system which in turn, negatively affects digestive processes. The body is programmed to switch off digestive processes when under stress, as the production of adrenalin takes place when the body is preparing for action not digestion.

BLACK TEA – contains the same stimulants as in coffee, though not in such high degrees. The main concern in drinking a strong tea brew regularly is that it provides excessive levels of tannic acid. Tannic acid binds beneficial alkaline minerals from your diet, making them unavailable for the body to use. The alkaline minerals – calcium and magnesium are particularly affected, without magnesium your body cannot digest food and without calcium your skeletal system will suffer. Both nutrients are required for cardiovascular function and many other body functions, in particular magnesium for regulating the sodium/potassium pump for cellular electrolyte balance for the nervous system.

SUGAR – has no nutritive value, is acid forming and is very destructive in every part of the body. It stimulates the adrenal glands, directly raises blood sugar levels and is addictive. With regular intake of sugar, your B vitamins and zinc can become depleted, these nutrients are needed to control stress, to produce stomach acid, sex hormones, balance blood sugar and for many other metabolic processes. Refined sugar or any type of sugar interferes with conversion of essential fats from the diet, it also suppresses the white blood cell count – your immune system army which protects you from infection and disease.

You can imagine the effect in the gut – sugar feeds bugs, not just the healthy ones but the bad colonies of organisms that run riot, multiplying and causing digestive havoc. This situation is perfect for other opportunistic bugs to get a hold and for you to end up with fungal overgrowth, parasitic or bacterial infections, with symptoms of bloating, painful cramps or food intolerance. This in turn can lead to chronic digestive disorders.

SLEEP DEPRIVATION – under these circumstances, the body tissues have difficulty renewing cells efficiently. Growth, detoxification and cell renewal takes place when the body sleeps. Your sleep body clock controlled by hormones is synchronized with your gut body clock, which is in tune with digestion. Poor sleep patterns affect digestion and hormonal balance.

STRESS – relentless stress through a busy lifestyle can cause untold damage throughout your body. As digestive processes switch off under stress – this is a biological function of ancient man when energy was needed for hunting; continued stress can cause the onset of digestive complaints. You cannot digest well if you are racing around and not relaxing enough to eat and digest your meals. When the body is at rest, digestive processes function best. If nutrients are used up in the stress cycle, then there is a deficit for digestive function.

A survey with 2,000 participants which studied the eating habits of adults in Britain, found that a quarter of people in the UK grab snacks to survive as opposed to eating three square meals a day and half of the population eat meals in front of the TV or computer.[3] This trend is obviously not conducive to healthy digestive function. It is stressful for your digestive system. For your health – the most important daily function you will ever perform is the process of a healthy eating pattern. Enjoying choosing delicious food, cooking dishes that nourish all the senses, and taking that opportunity to relax and re-charge your batteries.

YOUR BODY IS COMPOSED OF ELEMENTS DERIVED FROM YOUR FOOD

99% of the human body mass is made up of six main elements – oxygen, carbon, hydrogen, nitrogen, calcium, phosphorus. These and numerous other elements including potassium, sulphur, sodium, chlorine, magnesium, iron, manganese, zinc, copper, selenium and iodine, we derive from our diet. Food contains dozens of elements and trace elements that preserve health by supporting all the *'wear and tear'* processes that the human body is constantly undergoing. It is estimated that the body is comprised of approximately 70% water, so becoming dehydrated can have serious consequences.

The human body contains trillions of cells each having a certain lifespan, every organ has its own repair programme. Diet is a major factor in determining how successful these processes are in doing the job they are designed for. The human body has an amazing self-healing ability, a process of cell re-generation that can promote good health, providing the raw materials are to hand and the right conditions in place.

Your daily diet and lifestyle routine may cause small nutritional imbalances, but this may be of little significance and is usually a result of environmental factors, stress levels and precise quality of diet. Health problems however can start to manifest themselves when chronic nutrient deficiencies develop due to long-term poor dietary choices and imbalanced diet with a lifestyle incompatible with good health. The body is constantly renewing itself, sloughing off old cells and rebuilding new ones with the basic raw materials that are provided by your diet, if these are in short supply, cell renewal is compromised.

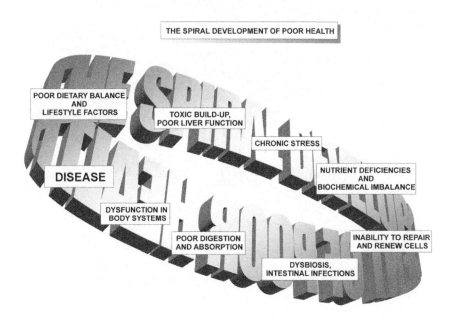

THE SPIRAL DEVELOPMENT OF POOR HEALTH

POOR DIETARY BALANCE, AND LIFESTYLE FACTORS

TOXIC BUILD-UP, POOR LIVER FUNCTION

CHRONIC STRESS

NUTRIENT DEFICIENCIES AND BIOCHEMICAL IMBALANCE

DISEASE

DYSFUNCTION IN BODY SYSTEMS

POOR DIGESTION AND ABSORPTION

INABILITY TO REPAIR AND RENEW CELLS

DYSBIOSIS, INTESTINAL INFECTIONS

THE TREE OF LIFE

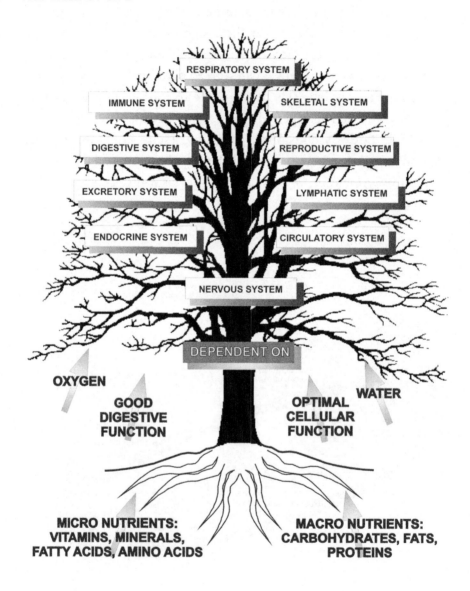

DID YOU KNOW?

- Your intestinal lining is replaced every four days
- Your body produces on average 2 litres of digestive juices daily
- Your immune army of white blood cells is replaced every week
- Oxygen carrying red blood cells are renewed every four months
- Your exterior skin is replaced monthly
- Your entire skeletal structure re-generates every three months
- Your liver re-generates at a phenomenal rate, in two months it can grow back to a healthy size following 70% surgical removal
- Your heart is the least regenerative organ, only half the cells get replaced in a lifespan
- Your brain cells last a lifetime[4]

Breaking-down, building-up, repair of cells is going on every second of life and these biochemical processes require an adequate and balanced level of carbohydrates, fat and protein, from the macro-nutrients and a balanced intake of micro-nutrients, vitamins, minerals, trace elements plus water. Your body requires dozens of nutrients daily – some essential such as vitamin C which the human body cannot synthesize and others non-essential which enable the body to combine and produce other nutrients. There are nine essential amino acids for cell building that must be present in the diet – Histadine, Isoleucine, Leucine, Lysine, Methionine, Phenylalanine, Threonine, Tryptophan and Valine.

The body has inborne systems of compensation to deal with poor dietary choices and toxic challenges to the body and will generally cope.[5] But when this situation becomes prolonged or other stresses present themselves, the body, which can be compared to a *'boat'* that has become top heavy – can start to falter in its functions and widespread nutritional deficiencies can develop, which in turn can lead to enzyme deficiency, low stomach acid and diminished reserves. As the immune system becomes challenged and dysbiosis in the gut develops, this precarious situation can escalate and tip the balance onto a slippery slope towards ill health.

Considering all the many factors that can lead to digestive disorders – the good news for you as a reader, is that chronic digestive health problems can be reversed or at least drastically improved given the right conditions. Even when a condition is advanced or requires surgery, there is always healing to be done, improvement to be made. The human body has an inbuilt ability to self-heal, to return the body to a state of equilibrium.

THE ROLE OF NUTRIENTS IN THE BODY

POTASSIUM	Works with sodium to help regulate the body's fluid balance, it helps keep heart rhythms normal, relaxes nerves and muscles after contraction. It is a main blood mineral, which together with sodium and chloride are known as electrolytes as they carry a small electrical charge. Magnesium regulates the sodium-potassium pump which governs the electrical activity in nerve cells. Potassium helps convert glucose for energy storage and release. It is also required by the thyroid gland to produce thyroxine which regulates metabolism
SODIUM	The main mineral found in the blood and body fluids, about 60% is in the fluid around the cells, 30% is in bones and the rest inside cells. Your body contains and needs salt to exist, in the right form from a sodium-rich diet. Both potassium and sodium are alkaline elements

ZINC	Involved in numerous enzyme functions, cell division, growth and repair, is particularly vital with vitamin C for building new skin. It is important for taste and smell, has anti-oxidant properties, and is required for immune system function. Zinc as a component of insulin is needed for blood sugar control, it is required in hundreds of biochemical reactions throughout the body and is one of the most important trace elements. You produce stomach acid for digesting protein with the aid of zinc and vitamin B6. Zinc is critical also for reproductive health
MANGANESE	Involved in glucose metabolism. It activates enzyme systems for body function and is required for skeletal development. It maintains sex hormone production, is involved in fat and carbohydrate metabolism and is also important for the nervous system and thyroid function
CHROMIUM	Works together with manganese to help control blood sugar levels. It regulates carbohydrate metabolism by enhancing insulin function
MOLYBDENUM	Important for many enzyme systems, it is involved in uric acid metabolism and helps to mobilise iron from storage sites in the body
MAGNESIUM	Essential for nerve and muscle function, for nervous system control, for converting carbohydrate into energy and for fat metabolism, it regulates heartbeat, helps maintain body temperature, strengthens blood vessels, regulates bone health, and is necessary for numerous enzyme activities. Both calcium and magnesium are alkaline elements

CALCIUM	Assists in blood clotting function, muscle contraction, heart and nerve function and maintenance of teeth and the skeletal system
PHOSPHORUS	85% of phosphorus is found in bones and teeth, bound with calcium. Both minerals compete for absorption in the intestines and certain foods containing oxalates and phytates can interfere with a healthy ratio by reducing absorption of calcium
COPPER	Is required for the formation of haemoglobin, your oxygen carrying molecule, it is also required for cell respiration, a process that releases energy. Collagen, part of the connective tissue in muscles and bone requires copper with vitamin C for cross linking and renewing structure. Copper is necessary for many enzyme systems, it also contributes to the integrity of the myelin sheath which covers nerves. Tyrosine an amino acid needs copper for its conversion to melanin, which gives hair and skin the colouring pigment. Copper helps nervous system function as it conducts electricity and assists with other metals, the electrical firing activity of our neurones
SELENIUM	As a trace element, it is only required in small amounts in the body. It acts as an antioxidant together with vitamins A, C, E, protecting cells from free radical damage which is explained in more detail in chapter 6
IRON	Approximately 60% of the body's iron is in the haemoglobin molecule in the blood, which carries oxygen through your body

VITAMIN A	Involved in health of eyesight, internal and external skin and immune function. With vitamins C, E and selenium it performs a cell protective antioxidant function
VITAMIN B COMPLEX	Health of the nervous system, required for digestion, hormone regulation, health of skin, eyes, red blood cell production, for immune function, for healthy brain function, for energy production
VITAMIN C AND BIOFLAVONOIDS	Antioxidant role, essential for formation of skin, collagen structure in connective tissue, vital for healthy gums, vision, and integrity of vascular system. It has a major role in supporting function of the immune system by destroying germs and bugs
VITAMIN E	Protects health and function of the Nervous System, supporting healthy skin and hormonal balance, it is a co-factor for selenium
VITAMIN D	Regulates the calcium/phosphorus ratio for bone and teeth formation, it also supports healthy immune function
VITAMIN K	Important for blood clotting function. Healthy gut bacteria also contribute to vitamin K production together with B vitamins within the body

Recommended dietary allowances (RDA) have not changed since the Second World War, they indicate the level of nutrients required to avoid deficiency diseases. The ideal daily levels in fact for optimal health in individuals are much higher than these figures. The RDA for vitamin C is 30mg, however the optimum level in fact for optimum nutrition is more in the region of 1,000mg plus. The RDA for B vitamins range from 1 – 18mg, but the optimum level is between 50 – 100mg.

Certain groups in the population have higher requirements for nutrients than others: the elderly, the sick or hospitalised, babies, young children, teenagers, pregnant mothers or those engaging in extreme sports or heavy manual labour.

A report by Marie Woolf, the Political Editor of *The Independent's* Health & Wellbeing section, back in 2007, said there were alarming levels of malnutrition in the British public, especially in hospital patients in all age groups. This is hardly surprising when the nation is trying to nourish itself with fast, long shelf-life convenience foods, often devoid of nutrients but containing a range of food additives from artificial colouring, emulsifiers, preservatives, flavourings – a whole toxic mix of chemicals that replace or disturb the nutrients in food.

With yearly rising figures of over 80,000 chemicals used in food production, packaging and homecare products industries, is it any wonder that nutritional deficiencies and toxic induced ill health exists in the affluent Western societies.[6]

Independent studies show that the nutritional content of food has fallen dramatically over the past few decades.

Paul Anthony Taylor of *Doctor Rath Health Foundation* – stated recently that 'vitamin and mineral deficiencies in the general population are quite widespread in Europe'.

HEALTH PROBLEMS LINKED TO NUTRIENT DEFICIENCY

ESSENTIAL FATTY ACIDS	skin rashes, dry skin and eyes, nervous disorders, mental instability	scaling and eczema, hormonal complaints, poor concentration, cardiovascular health problems
VITAMIN A	mouth ulcers, dry flaky skin, diarrhoea, cataracts	acne, poor night vision, frequent colds and infections, dandruff
VITAMIN C	frequent colds or infections, low energy	easy bruising, bleeding gums
VITAMIN D	joint pains or stiffness, poor immune function, hair loss, muscle cramps	tooth decay, excessive perspiration, low energy
VITAMIN E	easy bruising, lack of sex drive, varicose veins	slow wound healing, exhaustion after light exercise
B VITAMINS	poor skin health, eczema, depression, bloodshot burning gritty eyes, nerve weakness, poor memory and concentration, poor hair condition, sensitive tongue, irritability, nervous disorders	dry scaly skin, cracked lips, insomnia, headaches, sore muscles, split nails, stress, nausea, PMT, poor appetite

CALCIUM AND MAGNESIUM	muscle cramps, high blood pressure, skeletal health problems, tooth decay	palpitations, insomnia, stress
IRON	pale skin, sore tongue, ridging on nails	anaemia, appetite loss
ZINC	loss of taste and smell, frequent infections, hormonal imbalance, digestive problems	white marks on fingernails, stretch marks on skin, acne, poor skin health, infertility
COPPER	hair loss, heart disorders	loss of pigmentation in skin and hair, anaemia
POTASSIUM	irregular heartbeat, insomnia, menstrual problems, tension	muscle spasms, twitches, tingling, fluid retention, anxiety, thyroid problems

THE FOUR POINT RECOVERY PLAN

The Four-Point Recovery plan listed in this book is designed to help reverse digestive disorders and allow a healing process to take place, but it does need a focused input from you, to comply with recommendations and avoid bad habits during treatment which will hinder any programme you are following. It outlines a distinct plan and protocol for reversing the symptoms of chronic digestive health problems, following four very simple measures that need to be set in place in order that the body may heal and return to good health.

- **Remove**
- **Replace**
- **Repair**
- **Restore**

A full explanation of these procedures that apply to the gut, and the steps necessary to put them in place is mentioned in chapter 6.

Digestive disorders develop initially as a direct result of poor diet and faulty lifestyle. Effectively speaking these conditions can be resolved by assessing and addressing the root cause of the symptoms, even when tissue damage has occurred.

By removing offending components in the diet, replacing missing elements, repairing the gut and restoring gut integrity and healthy microbial balance – digestive disorders can be successfully reversed.

YOUR HEALTH IN YOUR HANDS

It is your body; you know it best and you can be in control of what you take into your body and determine what level of toxin exposure your body will be exposed to. Taking this route of healthcare can give you satisfaction and fulfilment, it can inspire you to be compliant with recommendations, as you, with good advice, are starting the process of healing your own body instead of feeling helpless and lost and putting your body in other hands.

You are no longer feeling out of control and dependant on medical advice that is not working for you. You have the knowledge; you have the tools.

Remember the human body always strives to maintain equilibrium and is constantly evolving to keep you healthy. The trick in achieving this desired state is not to keep challenging your body systems to put up with faulty lifestyle, poor diet, lack of rest and high stress from your choice of modern lifestyle.

You have one body and quality of life is foremost, otherwise being sick and suffering digestive problems is not an enjoyable state to be in.

The right conditions, apart from a healthy well-balanced diet, should include, from the onset, a full understanding of how the body works, how the digestive system functions, which nutrients are necessary for digestion, absorption and utilisation of food and how energy is produced in the body. You need this energy from food to fuel your metabolism to fuel your digestive system.

Once armed with all the information, you can formulate a plan of action and although a determined effort is required to follow new unfamiliar guidelines, the benefits to be gained are worth all the effort.

> *'It is far more important to know what sort of person the disease has than what sort of disease the person has.'*
> Hippocrates 460 BC

The right conditions also involve treating the patient not the disease. The standard medical approach for chronic digestive disorders focuses on symptom management with drugs. Rarely, there are cases who may require surgery for severe intestinal damage or the disorder becomes an acute critical case instead of a chronic disorder. But the source or root cause of the symptoms are not standardly deemed important, nor is the concept generally accepted that one part of the body part is intrinsically linked to all other parts.

What affects one area of the body certainly has an effect throughout every other body system. Modern Medicine focuses on treatment of disease and cannot devote the time it requires to investigate the underlying root cause of symptoms or support the maintenance of good health.

Joseph Pizzorno Jr in his paper 'Clinical Decision Making – Functional Medicine in Perspective' states that "The Personalisation of Care achievable through the Functional Medicine approach is the only real solution to the crisis of chronic disease facing us today."[7]

Functional Medicine is gaining in popularity as the modality of choice for chronic disease. The depth of attention applied to a patient's symptomology and the practical applications for assessing and treating gut disorders is truly symbolic of 'treat the patient not the symptoms'.

It appears the medical profession are showing increased interest in applying for training in this area of healthcare.

NUTRITIONAL MEDICINE

Nutritional Therapy is a drug-free holistic natural approach to healthcare which also incorporates Functional Medicine. It treats symptoms of ill health at the cellular level, assessing all the complex biochemical functions, the role of nutrients in digestive processes, and their function within the cell. It addresses nutritional and biochemical imbalances that are known to be linked to symptoms of poor health.

Nutritional or biochemical imbalance is assessed with Functional Medicine laboratory tests. Nutritional Therapy is the ideal therapy for addressing all digestive health problems, no matter what the diagnosis is, as nutrients are involved in every process of digestive function, whether it's Vitamin B 6 and Zinc required for production of stomach acid or the B vitamins, magnesium, manganese, copper, iron, Vitamin C and CoQ10 required for carbohydrate, fat and protein digestion.

The use of selective nutrients to heal and improve health, is a natural process for the body to utilise as opposed to synthetic drugs, which in contrast, are foreign to body tissue. Your individual metabolism will determine how well you make use of a healthy diet. Fine tuning the sort of diet to suit your individual, biochemical make-up will enhance absorption and nutrient uptake.

FACTORS ASSESSED DURING
A NUTRITIONAL CONSULTATION:

- Medical history, presenting symptoms, sleep pattern, lifestyle, dietary habits
- Anti-nutrient factors, stimulants and stress
- Genetic and biochemical make-up and family history
- Digestive and immune function
- Nutritional balance, medications, fitness and exercise

WHAT IS OPTIMUM NUTRITION?

This is an ideal state when all nutrients necessary for human health are present in your daily diet acting as an insurance policy against disease and infection. It encourages healthy digestive function, good energy levels, a positive mood, good concentration and generally a feeling of fitness and well-being.

You may be aware of basic advice given to eat plenty of fruit, greens and to avoid sugar and sweets, however it is not only your choice of food that is important but the nutrients within the calories. It is the quality and balance within your diet not the quantity of calories that count. Look at the body as a finely tuned engine that needs the right food as fuel. It may get by on processed nutrient deficient food for occasional periods in time – but there is a limit to what the body can endure.

When body stores of nutritional reserves run low and immune function becomes challenged, the tolerance level can soon turn into intolerance, with body systems becoming dysfunctional and patterns of ill health developing.

The gut is the most prominent player in the field. By addressing at an early stage minor dysfunction in digestion, obvious signs that the body is not happy with the choice of fuel, recognising the cause and dealing with it – can avoid much future distress. Damaging effects on the body can start to accumulate when the body is exposed to environmental toxins, pollutants chlorine and possibly fluoride in the water supply, artificial additives in the food supply, food contamination from packaging materials,[8] intensive farming practices that produce nutrient deficient soils and toxic chemical residues in produce. All this, with added stresses of modern life, insufficient rest and sleep, can mean your health can start to suffer. Challenges on the body, that it simply cannot cope with.

Nutritional Therapists follow an orthomolecular approach to health care, the phrase first 'coined' in 1968 by Linus Pauling in his classical paper 'Orthomolecular Psychiatry' in the *Science* Journal, which emphasised the need to supply the right molecules or nutrients from diet for efficient biochemical function to maintain human health.

Far too little emphasis in the medical profession is put on nutrition and diet. The body is not sick due to lack of drugs, but it can be sick due to lack of dozens of nutrients that the body requires in the daily diet. Digestive disorders are fully preventable.

Poor lifestyle, diet, drugs, stress, environment and other factors can deplete the body's reserves of nutrients, deficiencies can then lead to body systems failing to function correctly, as the raw materials they require for efficient action become unavailable.

Dr Carl C. Pfeiffer in his excellent book *Mental and Elemental Nutrients* supported nutrition as preventative medicine and pioneered the therapeutic orthomolecular use of nutrients in mental health at the Brain Bio Centre, Princeton, New Jersey, USA.

He recognised the harmful effect of toxins, environmental pollutants and nutrient deficiencies in the human body. His studies and research with nutrients in place of drug therapy as treatment protocols – specifically in mental disease, showed some amazing positive results.

This highlights the fact that all body systems are intrinsically inter-connected and dependent on each other. All body systems work symbiotically together and never in isolation. So often a deficiency of one or two nutrients can negatively affect correct functioning of another. Nutrients always work with other nutrients as co-factors – vitamins or minerals or in combination with amino acids or fatty acids and trace elements.

A good example is with fatigue – to produce energy in the cell, you require nutrients, mainly B vitamins, magnesium, iron, CoQ10, vitamin C, manganese, sulphur and copper. If your diet lacks foods containing any of these nutrients, the body will struggle to produce energy. Like any living organisms or even non-living, such as a car – it requires the right fuel.

Depending on your own unique biochemical make-up, you will have individual requirements for nutrient levels to enable you to keep your own body fit and healthy. There are no two humans biochemically identical; even within families, every human is quite unique. Individuals also metabolise foods at different rates, certain categories of food, in a certain ratio of carbohydrates, fat and protein will suit some metabolic types but will not be well tolerated in others. There is not one diet that suits all, just as there is not one pill that will have identical effects in all humans. Having said that however, the diet should always be nutritionally balanced, but the ratios can be adjusted in tune with the requirements of the body. A nutritional consultation can assess the type of dietary balance best suited for you.

WHY SUFFER? YOU CAN HELP YOURSELF TO DIGESTIVE HEALTH

Opting in to a new regime and changing habits of a lifetime can never be easy, a new way of thinking that may not fall in with your current way of life. It may cause you conflicts with your family and friends or within the work place. This could be a great challenge for you, but always keep focused on the issue in hand. Often the thought is worse than the action. Take simple measures such as improving diet, avoiding stimulants, getting more exercise, sunshine and fresh air, chewing food properly, all this can bring positive results very quickly. Taking time to de-stress and relax whilst eating, changing destructive bad habits, getting more sleep and drinking plenty of pure water, can bring untold improvements to your health and well-being.

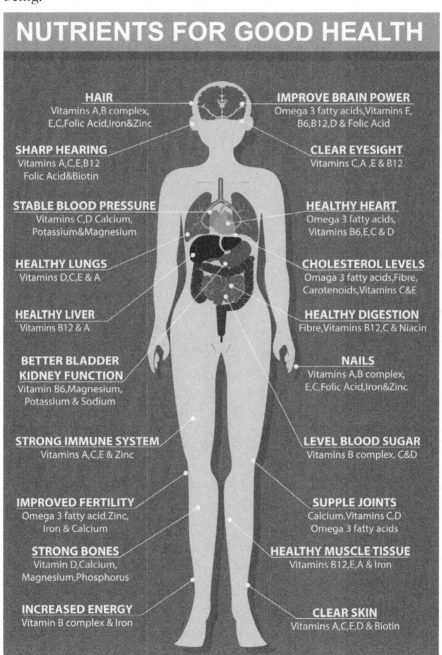

CHAPTER THREE

A Tour Through
the Intestinal Tract

'The wondrous world within.'
'Know thyself.'
Socrates 469 BC

The organs of digestion consist of your mouth, pharynx, oesophagus, stomach and your small and large intestine. The liver, pancreas and gallbladder are organs that aid in the chemical digestion of food.

THERE ARE FIVE STAGES OF DIGESTION:

- Ingestion   process of eating, taking food into the body

- Movement of food   passage of food through the gastrointestinal tract

- Digestion   breakdown of food by mechanical and chemical means

- Absorption   passage of digested food from the gastrointestinal tract into the cardiovascular and lymphatic systems for distribution to cells

- Elimination   removal of waste material from the process of eating

DIGESTION

When you eat your meals, the food is not in a form that can be used as an energy source within the cell.

The function of the digestive system is to digest and absorb your food. This takes place in a series of mechanical and chemical changes which breaks down your food, from a chemically complex form, into nutrients that are small enough to pass through the intestinal wall for transportation by the bloodstream into cells throughout the body.

MECHANICAL DIGESTION

The mechanical part of digestion consists of various movements of the gastrointestinal tract that aid the chemical breakdown of food.

Through thorough chewing, the food is mixed with saliva and the resulting food 'bolus' moves down the oesophagus by the act of swallowing into the stomach. Here smooth muscles of the stomach and the small intestine churn the food bolus, mixing it with enzyme secretions in gastric digestive juices, that are produced by cells along the intestinal tract.

The oesophagus does not produce enzymes, it secretes mucus to protect the gut lining and transports food to the stomach.

Food is pushed through the intestinal tract by peristalsis – muscular movements which contract and squeeze, in repeating wave-like motions.

The passage of food from the mouth to the stomach takes 4–8 seconds, liquids pass through in about one second. There is a sphincter (narrowing of the oesophagus) at the lower end of the oesophagus; this relaxes during swallowing, which allows the food bolus to enter the stomach. Contraction of the sphincter then takes place, to stop the acidic stomach contents from re-entering the lower oesophagus and irritating the oesophageal wall.

Reflux or heartburn can occur when the oesophageal sphincter lacks tone, fails to close properly or has delayed contraction.

When the sphincter fails to relax (during hurried meals for instance) the passage of food is impeded, and distension and discomfort can often mimic the intensity of cardiovascular chest pain.

There is a further sphincter (narrowing or valve) at the lower end of the stomach before the entrance to the small intestine, this is called the pyloric sphincter. Under control of muscular contraction, if this fails to relax, it can cause spasms and ingested food cannot easily pass into the small intestine; the resulting build-up of pressure can cause vomiting or discomfort.

The ileocecal-sphincter, a valve in the intestinal tract, guards the opening from the small intestine to the large intestine. It allows the digestive material to pass through and opens and closes during digestion.

In the case of chronic constipation, irritable bowel and other digestive disorders that affect the mechanical side of digestion, the action of this valve can become hindered, resulting in it only partially opening or closing. Subsequent distention, and soreness in this area, which lies between your belly button and your right hipbone can be very distressing. Often massaging the area with essential oils can relieve the pain but dealing internally with the cause of the problem is necessary to correct the dysfunction and heal the gut.

CHEMICAL DIGESTION

This is a series of chemical reactions by stomach acid and salivary, gastric, intestinal digestive enzymes, that break down the large macro-elements in food – the carbohydrate, fat and protein into smaller elements; the nutrients that are the vital part of your diet that nourishes your cells.

These elements are small enough to be readily absorbed through the walls of the intestinal tract into the blood and lymph capillaries and finally to be transported and utilised in the cells throughout your body.

After the intake of food, the first process of digestion begins in your mouth, with breakdown of carbohydrate by an enzyme called salivary amylase.

It is therefore important to chew food well to allow this enzyme to do its job. A test you can do to demonstrate this, is to chew a piece of plain bread thoroughly enough for the carbohydrate to release its sugar. This results from the action of the carbohydrate-splitting enzyme – salivary amylase. Slowly the food will be masticated into a sweet tasting material.

Chewing under stress and swallowing chunks of food can upset digestive processes further down the digestive tract, resulting in partially digested food which can start to ferment and cause irritation to the gut lining.

Slow wavelike motions, called peristalsis, project the food through the oesophagus and into the stomach, where protein digestion begins.

The secretion of your gastric juices in the stomach is regulated both by hormonal and nervous mechanisms. You may have heard the term butterflies in your stomach? Messages are quickly relayed from the brain to the stomach via the Autonomic Nervous System and can have an immediate effect on the digestibility of food.

Stress and reflexes from nerve impulses can inhibit gastric secretions.

This would be detrimental for your digestion as under these circumstances your digestive processes switch off, as your inbuilt physiological mechanisms 'prepare for battle'! We do not live in ancient times, but these mechanisms and hormonal reactions are still part of the modern human body and will be for ever more.

Here, in the stomach, chemical digestion takes place, where the food mixes with gastric juices, which contain hydrochloric acid, water and enzymes that break down and unravel the structure of the protein in your food.

You produce on average 1–2 litres of acidic gastric juices daily. The acidic environment of the stomach also acts as a guard against foreign microbes and infectious agents – protecting the body from attack. It is the first line of defence for your immune army of cells that protect against disease.

The body is finely tuned to digest protein in the acid conditions in the stomach but thereafter, as the food bolus progresses through the digestive tract, the environment becomes alkaline, due to the secretion of sodium bicarbonate from the pancreas; only then can digestion of all macro elements in your meal be completed in the small intestine, with the action of the pancreatic digestive enzymes.

STOMACH ACID FUNCTIONS:

- As a first line of defence, it prevents disease by destroying pathogenic organisms
- It breaks down protein into amino acids, providing building blocks for cell structures
- It aids pancreatic function by stimulating digestive enzyme production
- It facilitates the digestion and absorption of nutrients

When GPs are presented with heartburn, bloating or gastric reflux symptoms, it is commonly linked to signs of over production of stomach acid, and proton pump inhibitors PPIs, and other antacid medications are the medication of choice. These drugs reduce and in some cases over time, stop the production of stomach acid. A drastic action, as taking medication that interferes with protein digestion, can produce consequences throughout the body. The human body is designed to produce stomach acid, and in the less common cases of true over-production, alkaline mineral mediator options would be less harmful. Malabsorption and development of atrophic gastritis, have been implicated with the use of PPIs.[1]

Low stomach acid is, more often than not, the root cause of heartburn and reflux disorder. A recent 2017 study found it to be 'a surprising cause of indigestion' [2]. Clinical Nutritionists have known for years that Betaine Hydrochloride treatment for low stomach acid, has given positive results, especially for symptoms of indigestion, bloating and discomfort after eating.

Low stomach acid causes poor digestion of protein, protein can take much longer to digest than carbohydrate, if it is not fully broken down, it can sit in the stomach, and start to ferment from the sugars in the carbohydrate content of your meal. This then can give rise to a burning sensation and the stomach contents can leak back up into the oesophagus.

Low stomach acid is termed Hypochlorhydria, absence of stomach acid is called Achlorhydria and excessive stomach acid – Hyperchlorhydria. Low stomach acid is much more common than recognised. However, gastritis can be a result of both high and low stomach acid, so professional diagnosis is to be advised.

Through excessive long-term use of antacid medication, and subsequent inflammation caused by poor breakdown of food, the stomach mucosal lining can atrophy; this damaged gastric cell structure cannot then perform the task of producing stomach acid.

Reduced gastric secretions can result from many single or accumulative factors and can lead to a variety of chronic health problems.[3] There are studies that show gastric secretion declines with age, this obviously is dependent on genetic, lifestyle and dietary factors, however it is a fact you need to bear in mind, as with the process of ageing, nutrients are not so well absorbed, it is then even more important to lead a healthy lifestyle, and choose a supportive diet that nourishes the body.[4]

CAUSES OF LOW STOMACH ACID:

- Poor dietary choices with lack of nutrients, especially vitamin B6 and zinc required for stomach acid production
- Chronic stress and trauma
- The use of medications that interfere with digestive processes. NSAIDs – non-steroidal anti-inflammatories, PPIs – proton pump inhibitors, antibiotics. All, have a negative effect on stomach acid levels
- Ageing. A completely normal process of life, when all systems reduce in function
- Infections in the gastrointestinal tract

When stomach acid is low or absent, there is a higher risk of infection and vitamin B12 and iron absorption is reduced, these deficiencies can then lead to further health problems.

EFFECTS OF LOW STOMACH ACID:

- Maldigestion and malabsorption of nutrients
- Nutritional deficiencies. Deficiencies of calcium, magnesium, iron, selenium. zinc, copper and vitamin B12
- A risk of SIBO, small intestinal bacterial overgrowth
- Anaemia from poor iron absorption, pernicious anaemia from poor B12 absorption
- A risk of GERD, gastroesophageal reflux disease
- Increased gut permeability, a leaky gut
- Gastritis, colitis
- Food allergies and intolerance

- Auto-immune diseases
- Amino acid deficiency

So, what signs should you look for if you suspect you may have low stomach acid? Poor protein digestion due to low stomach acid leads to amino acid deficiency and can give rise to a multitude of symptoms. Protein is required for healthy skin, hair and nails, and to produce collagen, the most important structural protein in the human body.

Collagen is the 'cement' in your skin, the gel-like structure that holds teeth, bones, blood vessels and skin in place, binding together the cells in the body. When tissues and cells break down but cannot be efficiently renewed, with amino acids – the building blocks from protein, then body structure begins to fail.

SIGNS OF LOW STOMACH ACID:

- Bloating, flatulence, a rumbly tummy
- A feeling of fullness after eating a moderate portion meal, as if the meal is not being fully digested. An achy pain which is worse after eating
- Poor appetite, anaemia, fatigue. Muscles cramps in legs and feet, muscle wasting
- Poor nail health, ridging both vertical and horizontal, peeling and flaking nails
- Poor hair quality, rosacea, red patches on cheeks, burning mouth or tongue
- Gastrointestinal infections, burning, pain, cramping discomfort in gastric region
- Odorous mucus containing stools. Undigested food matter seen in stools. Diarrhoea
- Sensitivity to food – particularly protein
- Skin conditions, psoriasis, flaking, wrinkled dry skin

If you are still unclear whether your stomach acid levels are normal, there is a method at home to help determine stomach acid sufficiency.

Take ¼ of a teaspoon of bicarbonate of soda in ¼ cup of water, on an empty stomach. As the stomach acid reacts with the alkaline bicarbonate, it releases gas, within a few minutes you should burp. If there is no or little reaction, it is likely you have low stomach acid.

What to do if this is the case?

Take one betaine hydrochloride capsule (or betaine hydrochloride and pepsin) in the middle of your main protein-based meal. (This can be bought through any health shop.) If the result causes a burning sensation, then the chances are your stomach acid level is normal. If you feel no reaction but a comfortable feeling of digesting the meal, then the likelihood is, that your stomach acid may not be at an optimal level and you need HCL supplementation for a few months or longer. This can be taken, together with digestive enzymes as a long-term aid to digestion; plant enzymes will re-cycle in the body and help to improve your own production in time. Often, these measures can be found to resolve symptoms of digestive disorders without any further action required.

BENEFICIAL FOODS FOR LOW STOMACH ACID:

Fermented dairy and fermented vegetables such as sauerkraut. Digestive 'bitters' which stimulate the secretion of digestive juices – artichokes, dandelion, chicory. Apple cider vinegar and lemon juice.

There is a laboratory test available for assessment of gastric acid, this is mentioned in the resources section at the back of the book.

Low stomach acid can lead to tissue acidity. Protein has an acid ash after digestion. If incompletely broken down in the stomach, the acid from putrefying protein can leach through a damaged gut lining into the bloodstream.

The consequence of this, is a change in the acid/alkaline balance in cells. As acidic conditions worsen, the body will take alkaline minerals from bones and storage sites – calcium, magnesium, potassium and sodium, to help 'buffer' and reduce the acidity. Ultimately, this cascade of events can lead to osteoporosis, increased bone fractures, increased risk of cardiovascular disease and neurodegenerative conditions.

Eating under conditions where you are nervous, upset or anxious can affect stomach acid levels, causing gastrointestinal disturbances by disrupting digestive processes. Should this happen on a regular basis, partially digested food can remain too long in the intestinal tract causing bacterial overgrowth SIBO (small intestinal bacterial overgrowth) and increase the risk of heartburn or dyspepsia. A research study on 6,834 students, found a prevalence of reflux esophagitis GERD (gastro-oesophageal reflux disorder), associated with stress and the level of severity directly correlated with the degree of stress.[5]

Having emotional, mood and mind issues are usually linked to imbalanced body biochemistry. The supply of nutrients from your diet is not matching your needs. Orthomolecular therapy – the phrase used by Nobel Prize Winner Linus Pauling, meaning the use of the right nutrients for the treatment of disease, is a therapy practised by Clinical Nutritionists who focus on supplying your cells with the correct balance of nutrients.

Researchers found that anxiety and depression can also affect digestive function, and increase occurrence of GERD, causing some individuals difficulty in leading a normal lifestyle.[6]

Any form of body or mind stress can affect the digestive system. It is a vicious circle, with stress causing digestive problems and digestive problems causing stress. Dealing with the underlying cause of emotional or mental stress will help resolve these problems.

BASIC DIGESTIVE ENZYMES:

- Salivary amylase initially breaks down carbohydrate in the mouth, completion occurs with amylase in the small intestine
- Pepsin breaks down protein in the stomach
- Pancreatic proteases break down protein in the small intestine
- Trypsin and chymotrypsin produced by the pancreas break down protein in the intestine
- Lipase produced by the pancreas breaks down fats with the aid of bile salts
- In the small intestine – maltase, sucrase, lactase break down maltose, sucrose and lactose sugars in the diet

Peristalsis – muscular contractions in the wall of the gastrointestinal tract, propels the food through the intestinal tract, the contractions are stronger in the oesophagus and stomach region and weaker in the small intestine, the site of nutrient absorption.

Enzyme secretions which are produced by cells along the gastrointestinal tract then break down the food chemically. The small intestine is a tube over 6 metres in length. Food remains in the small intestine for a longer period of between three and five hours, where segmentation takes place. This is a localised contraction that mixes the food with digestive juices and brings the small particles of digested material into contact with the gut mucosal lining for absorption.

The result of all digestive processes ensures that your protein has turned into amino acids to be used for building blocks for new cells, your fats have been processed to fatty acids and glycerol to be used in cell metabolism and for structure of your new cell membranes and your carbohydrates have been turned into glucose, which is used as your energy source.

The fat is broken down in the intestinal area not only by lipase but is aided with emulsification action from bile salts, which are injected by the gallbladder into the small intestine, the gallbladder is a storage site for bile which is produced in the liver.

Imagine if you were suffering from some form of skin condition, which involved constant shedding of old skin cells. New cells need to replace the old, renewal is constantly taking place, and for this to happen you need plenty of amino acids from protein and fatty acids from fat in your diet, together with many different nutrients involved in skin health.

With these nutrients as material, your body will build new cells with the help of glucose from carbohydrates in your diet, used as the cell's energy source. If digestion is poor and your food is not fully digested, you could become seriously depleted in nutrient levels and this would hamper renewal of cells.

MAIN DIGESTIVE HORMONES:

Digestive hormones are chemical messengers which regulate the digestive processes

- Ghrelin, produced in the stomach, controls appetite by telling the brain when to eat
- Leptin is the main 'satiety hormone' that regulates when the body should stop eating
- Gastrin, produced in the stomach, stimulates release of the gastric juices
- Secretin, produced in the small intestine, stimulates the pancreas to produce sodium bicarbonate and the liver to produce bile
- Cholecystokinin, produced in the small intestine, reduces appetite and stimulates release of pancreatic digestive enzymes and bile from the gallbladder
- Gastric Inhibiting Peptide, produced in the small intestine, decreases stomach churning and slows stomach emptying
- Motilin, produced in the small intestine, increases gut motility and stimulates production of pepsin, required for protein digestion

A regular eating pattern is required for optimal digestive function. If you eat at all odd hours, your digestive body clock and sensitive digestive hormones will become dysregulated and out of order. This can be a contributory factor to the onset of chronic digestive disorders.

The human body consists of trillions of cells all of which need energy to undertake the myriad of functions necessary in keeping the body healthy. Their energy source comes from food, not just any category of modern day food, but a quality well-balanced, nutritious chemical-free diet. The nutrients are needed for healthy metabolism and should not be combined with man-made synthetic chemicals which have no role in the human body.

Cells in your body do not thrive well when presented with a cocktail of 'foreign material' in the form of food additives, a diet of processed food, seriously lacking in all the nutrients required for good health and numerous designer foods laden with chemicals that enhance marketing – it's like trying to run a car on lemonade.

The centre of your cell is called the nucleus, this is surrounded by the cytoplasm; where hundreds of chemical reactions take place every second of your life. Under the control of physical and biochemical functions in the human body, this activity is referred to as your metabolism.

Your basal metabolism, that refers to the sum of all chemical reactions that take place when the body is at rest involves:

Respiration, circulation, digestion, excretion, secretion, synthesis of special substances, maintenance of body temperature and growth and repair of all cells.

All these reactions in body systems require a top-quality diet, if you want to keep fit and avoid ill health and disease. Healthy metabolic function and support for cell renewal, that takes place continuously throughout your body, requires some major attention to your dietary choices without becoming fanatical. Your body deserves at least the basics and ideally a whole lot more. This means a regular daily intake of balanced macro nutrients – carbohydrate, fat and protein, which are broken down into all the various micro-elements; vitamins, minerals, fatty acids, amino acids and sugars to support energy needs and supply the building materials to maintain human life.

ABSORPTION

Is the process by which nutrients pass through the intestinal wall into the bloodstream to be taken off to your cells for all the multiple metabolic functions which take place in order to keep healthy. Within 3–5 hours after you have eaten your meal, the body has the task of breaking down your food and absorbing all the nutrients required for human health.

The stomach absorbs water, electrolytes (sodium, potassium) and additionally, if in the system, drugs and alcohol, which brings the liver detoxification pathways into action.

The absorption area in your small intestine is covered with tiny finger-like projections called 'villi', which facilitate the process of absorption. In coeliac disease, these 'villi' can become flattened and damaged, mainly through food intolerance related to gluten containing grains.

The resulting malabsorption of nutrients can only be corrected by strict adherence to a gluten-free diet. It is possible, sometimes, to re-generate these 'villi' and heal the intestinal lining.

In 'leaky gut' syndrome, similar damage can exist, but to a lesser degree. The main problem lies in the 'tight junctions' between intestinal cells becoming 'leaky' and more permeable, allowing undigested matter into the bloodstream. The tight junctions in the intestinal lining regulate the rate of absorption of nutrients from the diet.

Substances get in and out of cells, the process of absorption, by diffusion or active transportation. Intestinal cells take up certain substances such as nutrients from your food and transport them across the cell surface membrane into the bloodstream for transportation throughout the body.

With an unhealthy gut lining, such as in leaky gut, nutrient absorption can be considerably reduced.

Nutritional deficiencies may then develop and body systems will struggle to function well.

ELIMINATION

The waste material left after the process of digestion is mostly undigested matter. It finally enters the large intestine for excretion. Some water, and salt absorption takes place. Mucus to lubricate and defend the gut lining against bacteria is produced.

When excess mucus is seen in the stools this can be an indication of damaging microbial infection or food intolerance. The body protects itself by producing mucus to safeguard tissues throughout the body. With sinus/glue ear/colds and coughs the production of mucus reflects microbial attack in the upper respiratory areas.

Further processing of the material, occurs in the large intestine – by the time the food waste has remained in the large intestine for 3–10 hours, it has become semi-solid. The final stage of elimination occurs through bacterial action, not by enzymes as in the small intestine. Water is re-absorbed and the remaining waste material is prepared by bacteria for elimination.

The bacteria ferment any remaining undigested carbohydrates (sugars) and in doing so, release gases – these gases create flatulence, so you can easily imagine a link with episodes of bloating and flatulence after eating cane sugar in any form. Toxins taken into the body will be excreted with the stools, once they are successfully metabolised by the liver.

The odour in the faeces is connected to the bacterial breakdown of remaining proteins, if the odour is offensive, there is a likelihood of incomplete protein breakdown, due to insufficient stomach acid and protein splitting enzymes.

The actual colour and consistency of the faecal matter is very relevant. The formation of your stools can indicate what sort of diet you are eating and how well you digest your food.

Compacted, dark stools, point to lack of fibre, essential fatty acids and fluid in the diet, often indicating a high meat intake, with low complex carbohydrates and very little alkaline forming foods such as fruit and green vegetables. Deficiencies of vitamin C and magnesium are likely.

Light coloured, loose stools, can indicate a lack of protein, and a diet too high in carbohydrates and sugars with reduced bile function and possible deficiencies of amino acids, calcium and vitamin D.

Peristaltic movements push the stools into the rectum, and this pressure stimulates your need to empty the bowels. The whole elimination process is linked to receptor messaging via hormones and nerve cells.

Achieving regular elimination at least once daily is a healthy aim. This can be in response to a meal or a warm drink but should never be activated with straining. If this is the case, there is clearly a need to investigate the content and balance of your food and liquid intake, what goes in is what comes out and it should take place with little effort.

The stools should be light brown, soft and easy to pass. Dark-brown/black compacted, hard stools need urgent attention as this can lead to toxic bowel syndrome, old material, hard to pass, favours microbial infestation and toxic build-up. It then gets re-absorbed back into the bloodstream, causing systemic ill-health throughout the body.

If the food intake is well balanced and stools are still difficult to pass, then lack of exercise, low intake of fluids, lack of vitamin C and magnesium, and stress levels need evaluating.

Magnesium helps muscle relaxation and peristaltic movement in the intestinal tract. Vitamin C can soften the stools considerably and the two nutrients together can work wonders in aiding regular elimination. Having said this, one should look to the basic cause of the problem and this will mostly be poor dietary balance and lack of fibre intake.

Vitamin C rich fruits and dark green leafy vegetables and whole grains for magnesium should be included in the diet.

EATING FOR PLEASURE, GOOD DIGESTION AND HEALTH

Consider and reflect on what goes on in your body after you have eaten your food. This is the end of your eating for pleasure activity, and few people give more thought as to what happens to the food they are eating. There is however, more to just eating food for pleasure and enjoyment. A well-balanced diet needs to be digested and absorbed well, it requires peace and quiet and stress-free time to achieve this, otherwise it is just an expensive activity, with little gain in health for your body. A poorly balanced fast food diet can be eaten for pleasure and regretted at leisure.

Eating only for pleasure, as in the case of enjoyment of junk food, processed foods and stimulants which upset body biochemistry, and not paying attention to the body's needs for nourishment, is in effect, short changing yourself in terms of health; each unhealthy meal eaten is an opportunity lost to nourish your body.

The process of eating is in fact the beginning of your eating for health phase. The perfect opportunity to choose your food wisely with health in mind, plan your meals, plan the whole eating experience, a meal to enjoy, and put this into regular practise.

Poor dietary choice and wrong food combinations, poor mastication, stress whilst eating, not giving your body the restful time it needs to digest efficiently, can all be a recipe for disaster, increasing the risk of digestive problems arising. Understanding the process of digestion can hopefully encourage good habits for mealtimes.

FACTORS THAT NEGATIVELY AFFECT DIGESTIVE PROCESSES:

- Not chewing food well, rushed meals
- Drinking water with meals which dilutes stomach acid causing

a change in pH levels
- Stressful conditions when eating
- Not taking time to sit in peace and quiet for digestion to take place
- Being de-hydrated
- Lack of stored nutrients, needed for digestion – magnesium, folic acid, zinc, vitamins B1, 2, 3, 5, 6, 12, biotin, copper, iron, vitamin C and CoQ10. Stomach acid is produced by adequate zinc and vitamin B6.
- Too much calcium in the diet with not enough magnesium (calcium contracts muscles, magnesium relaxes) – this is important in peristaltic movement
- Combining fizzy drinks with meals
- Eating exceedingly spicy food
- Eating carbohydrate desert too soon after a protein meal
- Eating very hot or ice-cold foods and drink

Enzyme activity in the intestinal tract during digestion of food works within tight temperature parameters; very hot or icy cold food and drinks cause digestive enzymes to switch off activity and digestive function is compromised.

Think about supermarket produce that has displayed fresh fruit and vegetables in the chilled foods section – destroying the vital lifeblood of the produce, which are the enzymes. The product then begins to degrade rapidly and has a shorter shelf life. Un-chilled fresh produce lasts twice as long. The same thing happens in the human body; digestive enzyme processes switch off, if the stomach is confronted with extreme fluctuations in temperature with ingested food and drink.

ENERGY PRODUCTION IN YOUR CELLS

The nutrients in food, having been transported and distributed to all cells in the body, then become active in energy production.

Energy is released in cells by a process called oxidation; a complex chain of chemical reactions aided by nutrients, oxygen and water. About 95% of energy released by the process of oxidation of food appears in the body as heat.

This energy given off is in the form of a substance called ATP – adenosine triphosphate, an energy unit which is used in the process of building new cells. ATP is used as an energy source, for muscular activity, movement, respiration, digestion, maintenance of body temperature, brain activity, growth and repair and all the other processes taking place in your metabolism.

Poor cellular energy production can be due to variable factors linked to nutrient deficiencies, de-hydration, and cellular toxicity. Nutrients required for the energy production Krebs cycle in the cell, are B vitamins 1, 2, 3, vitamin C, iron, copper and CoQ10.

THE GASTROINTESTINAL TRACT

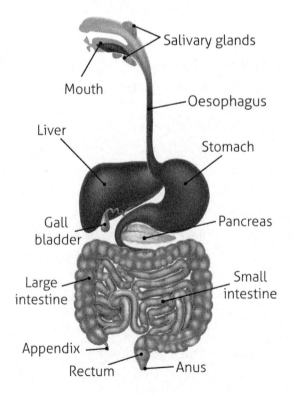

CHAPTER FOUR

Functional Medicine Laboratory Tests and Case Histories

'Illnesses do not come upon us out of the blue, they are developed from small daily sins against nature.'
Hippocrates 460 BC

FUNCTIONAL MEDICINE

Functional Medicine is currently being regarded as the medicine of the future and is gaining in popularity each year. A new model of healthcare that offers a totally different approach to dealing with the apparent world-wide epidemic of chronic disease.[1]

Chronic digestive disorders are a large part of this problem. The current healthcare systems are not able to deal with the enormous burden of chronic sickness, which is largely linked to food and lifestyle factors.

Environmental toxicity has increased, nutritional deficiencies across populations are on the rise and healthcare systems that manage acute and emergency care, face challenges with the steadily rising figures of chronic poor health. A different approach is required for individuals that can contribute personal support for their health problems. A systems-orientated personalised medicine model is ideally required for the treatment of chronic disease.[2]

The focus with current medical practice is on symptom management with drug therapy. This is appropriate for acute medical conditions but not appropriate for chronic disease. This model of healthcare fails to address the underlying causes of chronic ill health, as it is disease orientated, which focuses on the suppression of symptoms. A favourable flourishing situation for enormous pharmaceutical profits, but certainly not for the patient themselves. World-wide, there are thousands of deaths annually from drug related treatments.

The personalisation of care with drug-free solutions offered by Functional Medicine is the only real solution.

Natural medicine is under siege as pharmaceutical companies slander and discredit the value of natural supplements, botanicals and nutrients. All for the benefit of the enormous profit involved in drug marketing.

The situation is worse in the States but Europe suffers with similar problems due to drug and surgery orientated medical care. There are movements in the USA which are actively trying to introduce Nutritional Medicine into the medical training curriculum.

In the published fully referenced report 'Death by Medicine', authors state, "there is compelling evidence that medical systems of today frequently cause more harm than good".[3]

The following figures from the USA are staggering:

2.2 million people yearly have adverse reactions to prescribed drugs.

7.5 million people annually suffer unnecessary medical and surgical procedures.

8.9 million people are hospitalised annually.

A UK small study of 125 patients in London by Dr J Goffman was included in the report, who found over-investigation by MRI, CT, scans and X-rays contributed to 75% of all new cancers, together with inappropriate medication, poor diet and lifestyle factors.

90% of scans recommended produced negative results but achieved a high profit potential.

The most stunning statistic stated in this report, is that there are approximately 783,936 deaths in the US annually from conventional medicine, this in an age where vitamins are reported as being dangerous! Clearly there is something wrong in this approach and every reason for choosing to seek a non-harmful, non-invasive, gentle, in-tune with nature alternative. Avoiding medication for chronic digestive disorders is the best thing you can do for your body You have nothing to lose and a whole lot to gain.

Instead of achieving improvement and being cured of chronic disease through natural means, patients are usually offered medication or some cases surgery, for health problems that can be addressed purely by drug-free nutritional medicine and dietary and lifestyle changes.

With all serious or worrying health problems however, it is always advisable to seek a correct diagnosis from your doctor, regardless which route of treatment you may choose. You are not duty bound to accept treatment but for all serious health problems, professional advice is required.

Functional Medicine shifts the focus of care from suppression of symptoms to evaluation of diet and lifestyle. It addresses and treats the underlying root cause of chronic disease. It aims to identify, using the latest scientific advances in test procedures, biochemical imbalance in body systems.

With a patient centred approach, it offers a personalised system of care, that looks at the body holistically, instead of just the isolated symptoms or in a compartmentalised fashion.

There are strengths and failings in current health care systems, but the Functional Medicine model would solve many problems in easing the burden of management for chronic health conditions, which have been found in clinical practice to respond best to dietary and lifestyle interventions.

The practice of Functional Medicine, recognises the individuality and uniqueness of each person's biochemical and genetic make-up, and addresses this in their personalised approach to treatment and healing.

Functional Medicine is a unique system, in that it investigates every aspect of your well-being: interactions with the environment, influences from diet and lifestyle, gastrointestinal health, the microbiome, stress levels, sleep and relaxation patterns, toxic load, liver and digestive function, genetic tendencies, nutritional and biochemical balance.

SUMMARY

Functional and Nutritional Medicine is the treatment of choice for all types of chronic digestive disorders, it is clinically proven to bring lasting positive results. It will offer you peace of mind that you are receiving focused attention to every aspect of investigation concerning your health problem.

This approach works on the guidelines, that consultation and treatment is a partnership between practitioner and patient, encouraging you to take responsibility for your own health, to learn how to judge your own symptoms, monitor progress rather than being a submissive receiver of drug therapy that nobody, not even drug manufacturers can predict will cure or even give a healthy outcome in your individual body.

In Functional Medicine, nutritional and botanical supplementation does not replace medication in a fashion that mimics drugs; nutrients are used therapeutically to treat biochemical imbalances identified on test procedures, together with all the many other recommendations, concerning diet and lifestyle adjustments necessary for the body to heal itself. Botanicals enhance health of the gut, work in tune with nature and help to maintain microbial balance.

The treatment plans are not designed for long-term application to manage symptoms but constitute an action plan to put in place. These are measures that enable the body to reverse symptoms of poor health and help return the body to a state of good health. This approach focuses on your specific symptoms and the link to biochemical and nutritional dysfunction or imbalance. Treatment, of which you play a large part, is designed to help reverse all the damage and disruption to body systems that may have occurred over time. It puts therefore the whole balance of control firmly back in your hands – it is a partnership with nature.

WHAT IS METABOLIC TYPING?

Metabolic typing provides a method for identifying the best diet that suits your individual body chemistry, it follows the guidelines for individualised, finely-tuned nutritional interventions to ensure correct dietary balance and good digestion.[4]

Metabolically and biochemically every human on earth is completely unique. There are no two humans totally alike, even within families. Shapes and size of organs vary considerably as does individual biochemistry. Food can have virtually opposite effects or influences in different types of metabolism in various individuals.

Foods that energise and keep one person healthy, can cause fatigue and poor health in another. Eskimos, tribes in Africa, Aboriginals, Amazonian Indians would be eating vastly different diets to Europeans who have mixed and mingled genetically over centuries.

People also process and metabolise foods at different rates, and this is influenced by genetic make-up mainly but also by lifestyle and environmental factors.[5]

William Wolcott Nutritionist, Frances Pottenger MD and William Kelley DDS found in 1996 that some individuals broke down food with dominant influence from the oxidative system – the rate you burn off food for energy and others with dominant influence from the autonomic nervous system.

In fact, there are quite probably many variables in any category, but the practise does prove the point, that foods have different effects in different individuals. Some people feel extremely sluggish and inactive on higher protein and fat, others thrive on it. A high carbohydrate, fruit, vegetable, grain diet, with a little protein energises some individuals and makes others feel under the weather and unable to perform.

Knowing your body and noting reactions to certain meals with different balances of protein, carbohydrate and fat, can give you a guiding clue, on choosing the correct balance for your body type. Although sounding confusing, it can be beneficial to listen to your body and how it reacts to certain food categories.

If you are often hungry, not satisfied after eating, have sugar cravings, then your dietary balance is not in order. You may require more complex (unprocessed) carbohydrates to store glucose more efficiently, and more protein and healthy fat in a heavier diet to stabilise your metabolism, balance your hormones and help convert your food to energy.

If you lack energy, are unable to concentrate and feel lethargic after your meals, then you probably require less protein and fat in the diet which take longer to digest and to increase more energising carbohydrates – fresh fruit, vegetables and salad items in a lighter diet.

Children often fail to get the right balance of nutrient intake, surviving on quick sugar fixes which causes irritability, hyperactive behaviour and inability to concentrate and behave. Due to rapid growth, children need a high protein diet with plenty of healthy fats and fruit, vegetables and complex wholegrains to supply reserves for energy needs.

Your body is programmed to be healthy, if you are not, then two things need addressing. Are you eating a poor diet with junk food and stimulants? and is your ratio of the macro elements – carbohydrates, protein, fat correct for your body type? Provide the body with the raw materials in the right balance and the body will do the rest. This may take some experimentation but is easy to achieve.

CHECK YOUR CARBOHYDRATE/FAT/PROTEIN BALANCE

First ensure all carbohydrates, protein and fat are in their healthiest form, refer to the 'Recommendations for a healthy diet' in chapter 5.

Have a week of fruit, vegetables, salads, wholegrains, nuts and seeds, with a small amount of protein and animal fat, and see how you feel.

Breakfast example – fresh fruit, nuts, seeds, wholegrains with a little fruit juice and yoghurt.

The following week, base meals on a higher level of protein and animal fat, at each meal the same amount of vegetables but less fruit intake and lower intake of grains.

Breakfast example – yoghurt with some oats and blueberries, boiled or scrambled egg with mushrooms, or healthy cooked fish and meat options.

Given time you should be able to work out your body's reaction to a change of ratio between carbohydrate, protein and fat. Your aim is to feel energised and not to experience sugar cravings.

THE OXIDATIVE LEVEL – the rate you burn off food for energy

Some people burn food and nutrients too slowly and some burn them far too quickly. This action is determined by your genetic make-up and environmental factors.

A fast oxidiser with acidic tendencies in body tissues, burns off food at a faster rate than a slow oxidiser with more alkaline tendencies.

The fast oxidiser may crave salt, which being alkaline can offset acidic conditions. Individuals may be prone to indigestion, heartburn, insomnia, stress, diarrhoea, digestive problems, irritability, high blood pressure, arthritis or inflammation, have high energy output and are quite demanding types.

Conversely an alkaline slow oxidiser type may crave sugar and carbohydrates to boost energy levels, be prone to constipation, respiratory health problems, irregular heartbeat, lethargy, chronic fatigue, low blood sugar and allergies. A cautious and 'slow to anger' type.

Foods that suit a stressed fast oxidiser, are foods that take longer to digest and contain more fat. It is a richer, fattier 'heavier' diet that slows the metabolism down and de-stresses an over active individual with increased protein, essential and saturated fats. All food choices should be chosen with health in mind. If cardiovascular disease exists or blood fat disturbance is evident, there are essential fats to be recommended and saturated fats to be avoided. In this instance low fat protein would be recommended. Practitioner advice is then always recommended to ensure correct dietary procedures.

Foods that suit a slow oxidiser, are found in a lighter diet with plenty of fruit and vegetables, and grains for energy but only light protein – fish, chicken and lower fat, so that the body remains energised.

THE AUTONOMIC NERVOUS SYSTEM (ANS) – the main system in the body that regulates your metabolism.

Nutrients play a vital role in keeping the ANS in balance.

The Autonomic Nervous System is divided into two sides; the sympathetic and parasympathetic branches.

The sympathetic side is the 'fight or flight' adrenalin rush, all action ready, 'switch off digestion' mode, commonly experienced in the fast oxidiser. Stomach secretions for digestion decrease.

The parasympathetic side is when the body returns to normal homeostatic balance, or 'rest and digest' mode, commonly experienced by a slow oxidiser. Stomach secretions for digestion increase.

The hormones involved in these actions are under automatic involuntary action. In other words, you will not be aware of the action, but you will be aware of the effect of the action.

These two mechanisms should be well balanced; if there is dominance in any one branch, digestive function will be affected.

Chronic stress and manic hurried meals will switch on your sympathetic action and switch off your digestion.

You may have heard the expression 'one man's food is another man's poison'.

Wolcott, Pottenger and Kelley, demonstrated that the same foods and supplements could have opposite pH (acid/alkaline effects) in oxidative system dominant types as they would in autonomic nervous system dominant types.

The assessment was made after a 6-hour fast, with challenge drinks of glucose and protein.

Monitoring of urine, saliva pH and blood glucose levels over a period of two hours gave an indication of the variable outcomes, where the alkaline forming carbohydrate drink would cause acidity in some and alkalinity in others. The protein challenge had similar effects.

At a pH of 7.46, you digest, absorb and utilise food optimally. Your body is designed to function best under more alkaline conditions.

SUMMARY

The whole purpose of metabolic typing, is to see which type of diet is better suited to the individual. Either a lighter carbohydrate rich diet or a heavier protein rich diet, or combination of the two, and which types of food may have a detrimental effect because of your individual biochemical make-up.

It would not be recommended to rely on Metabolic Typing solely as a means for treating chronic digestive complaints, it is a therapy that may be considered, in a simplified version, in addition to Nutritional and Functional Medicine.

A Clinical Nutritionist or Functional Medical Practitioner can assess chronic digestive disorders comprehensively and effectively with laboratory analysis.

PART I

FUNCTIONAL MEDICINE LABORATORY TESTS

Specific Biochemical Diagnostic tests through specialised laboratories are used to assess and analyse the underlying cause of symptoms of ill health.

A list of some laboratories offering these tests will be found in the resources section at the back of the book.

The extensive range includes Gastrointestinal, Immunology, Endocrinology, Metabolic, Genetic and Nutritional Profiles which are all highly comprehensive and clinically valuable for practitioners. The information gained, pinpoints areas linked to the underlying cause of the health problem.

We will be focusing on the nutritional and gastrointestinal profiles, which will be explained in the context of case history studies from my personal practice. These tests are invaluable for assessing chronic digestive disorders.

TESTS LIKELY TO BE RECOMMENDED
FOR DIGESTIVE DISORDERS:

COMPREHENSIVE DIGESTIVE STOOL ANALYSIS (CDSA)

This test evaluates digestion, absorption, gut flora and inflammatory markers.

The Profile is indicated for all chronic digestive disorders.

COMPREHENSIVE DIGESTIVE
STOOL ANALYSIS + PARASITOLOGY (CDSA/P)

This test includes all the evaluation above but in addition tests for parasites using microscopic examination.

This Profile is likely to be recommended when a patient presents with irritable bowel syndrome (IBS) or colitis, diverticulitis, or any symptoms that indicate parasite infestation.

COMPREHENSIVE DIGESTIVE STOOL ANALYSIS 2.0 (CDSA2.0)

This test offers all the above evaluations but adds in risk assessment for colorectal cancer, differential diagnosis between IBS and IBD (inflammatory bowel disease), plus an assessment for exocrine pancreatic function (digestive enzyme) assessment.

This Profile is indicated for all chronic digestive disorders, acute bowel change patterns, and for many systemic diseases, that will always involve the gut.

COMPREHENSIVE PARASITOLOGY (CP) (stool test)

This test assesses bacteriology, mycology (yeast), parasitology and infectious pathogens (capable of causing disease) in the gut.

The test can be useful when a patient experiences signs of microbial imbalance or overgrowth, tends to have good digestion, few upper gastric symptoms but problems in the lower abdominal area.

Further add-on tests can be included for Helicobacter Pylori and other pathogenic bacteria that may be suspect in the symptom analysis.

GI EFFECTS COMPREHENSIVE PROFILE (stool test)

This is an advanced test, which uses specific complex markers for the monitoring and management of gastrointestinal disease.

LEAKY GUT TEST (CYREX A a2) (serum blood test)

Irritation from many sources can contribute to increased permeability in the gastrointestinal mucosa (gut lining), fungi, parasites, viruses, bacteria, toxins brought in externally with the diet or produced internally from microbial activity and fermenting undigested food matter. (Information on leaky gut is discussed in chapter 1.)

The Intestinal Antigenic Permeability Screen, the leaky gut test measures health of barrier structures: occulin, zonulin and actomyosin, the components involved in degradation of tight junctions which regulate gut permeability.

LPS (Lipopolysaccharides) – large molecules consisting of a fat and a sugar, are also measured.

Results indicate whether there is damage to the tight junctions in the intestinal tract. Damage from toxic compounds, pathogenic bacteria and undesirable large molecules that 'leak' through the lining, can challenge the immune system and lead to systemic inflammation.

This comprehensive test can indicate both increased permeability (leaky gut) and decreased permeability in the gut (malabsorption of nutrients).

GUT PERMEABILITY PROFILE (urine test)

The test uses two sugar molecules lactulose and mannitol taken orally. The degree of permeability or malabsorption is reflected in urinary collection over a period of 6 hours.

THE GASTRO TEST (string test)

Indicates the stomach acid level, differentiating between no stomach acid (achlorhydria, and low stomach acid (hypochlorhydria).

SECRETORY IMMUNOGLOBULIN A (s IgA) (saliva test)

This is the main antibody found in mucosal secretions throughout the body. It protects the body from pathogenic organisms and food allergens. Deficiencies are common with poor diet and stressful lifestyles.

A suitable test for all dysfunction in the immune and digestive system. Low levels of this important antibody can lead to recurrent infections anywhere in the body, this leads to a higher risk of increased gut permeability and food intolerance.

CANDIDA ANTIBODY AND IMMUNOLOGY PROFILE (saliva)

Candida albicans is an opportunistic fungus, a common species of yeast. There are many more strains that can cause fungal overgrowth in the gut, leading to systemic overgrowth in what is known as its mycelial form.

This test can be useful, however fungal overgrowth is also covered in the CDSA stool tests, which are more comprehensive, indicating overall links to infection.

CANDIDA IgG (serum blood test)
An antibody test that evaluates systemic yeast overgrowth.

YEAST CULTURE (stool test)
Evaluates the concentration of yeast present.

HISTAMINE (urine test)
Measures the amount of histamine released from mast cells. An indicator of inflammation and immune function.

DAO ENZYME (blood test)
The importance of a histamine test for digestive disorders, is that histamine is implicated in allergy, food sensitivities and leaky gut syndrome.

It affects the nervous system, influences the immune response and the physiological function of the digestive system. Histamine has a normal role in the immune system by attracting white blood cells to an area of infection, helping the white army of cells that permanently patrol the body, on the look-out for pathogenic invaders.

In the case of injury, the reddening effect at the site is due to histamine, which aids immune function. Production is under homeostatic control and health problems only arise when the balance is compromised, causing over production of histamine, either by an inflammatory promoting diet, inability to tolerate fermented foods, high stress levels or enzyme deficiency.

Histamine is a chemical compound that can cause allergic reactions. It may influence mast cells, a type of white blood cell, found throughout the body and which are part of the immune system. Mast cells contain histamine and other chemicals that destroy foreign invaders by bursting and releasing the potent load. This causes the anaphylactic shock response, urticaria, asthma, hives and swelling.

Evidence was reviewed in this 2012 article, on whether mast cells initiated the process of inflammation of the bowel wall in inflammatory bowel disease. The researchers concluded that mast cells may participate in contributing to motility disturbances but may not initiate the actual inflammation in IBD.[6]

Excess flushing on skin, often seen in the facial region of certain high metabolic types of individuals following a meal or alcohol intake, is due to histamine production. It can be produced in excess when foods high in histamine are eaten and the body either lacks adequate level of the enzyme DAO (diamine oxidase) that breaks down histamine, the person has poor methylation, which processes histamine or there is a deficiency of alkalising nutrients which offsets the histamine.[7]

Histamine is also a neurotransmitter involved in brain function, it communicates important messages from the body to the brain.

HIGH HISTAMINE FOODS:
Citrus fruits, kiwi, lemon, limes, plums, cocoa, chocolate, papaya, some nuts, wheat, yeasted foods, all fermented foods – alcohol, sauerkraut, well-ripened cheese, vinegar, yoghurt, kefir, pickles, olives, cured meats, overly ripened foods, especially bananas.

LOW HISTAMINE FOODS:
Meat, fish, chicken, eggs, non-citric fruits, root vegetables, dark green leafy vegetables, yeast-free, wheat-free grains, milk and dairy, coconut, rice, oils and herbs.

THE METHYLATION LINK TO HISTAMINE
Methylation is a biochemical pathway that uses the transfer of methyl molecules from your food, containing one carbon atom and

three hydrogen atoms, for metabolic enzyme functions in the body that produce energy, renew cells, and influence anti-oxidant cell protection. Poor methylation, as already mentioned, can increase histamine levels.

Methyl groups are essential in our diet, to support the methylation process.

Foods that contain good levels of methyl groups, are sugar beet, prawns, shrimps, leafy green vegetables, citrus fruit, strawberries, fish, meat, milk and eggs.

The process is dependent on nutrients – methionine; an amino acid from protein which when methylated, decreases histamine, betaine, B vitamins, magnesium, calcium, magnesium and zinc. A diet rich in protein and fats aids this function as fatty acids and amino acids can be utilised in methylation.

The need for methyl groups in the diet increases when you are under stress, and under stress the body's need for B vitamins, vitamin C, calcium, magnesium and zinc increase.

In the excellent book *Mental and Elemental Elements* by Carl. C. Pfeiffer, MD, mention is made that the effects of high histamine, a recognised biochemical imbalance called 'Histadelia' responds well to calcium, zinc and methionine.

In my practice, zinc methionine and calcium gluconate brought promising results in offloading and lowering brain tissue histamine, in a combination with low histamine foods. It is important not to use the citrate form for the minerals which can elevate histamine levels. Vitamin C also has beneficial anti-histamine effects and is vital for the control of stress.

Pfeiffer emphasised in his research, that patients who were sensitive to wheat gluten were not high, but low in blood histamine, an effect called 'Histapenia'.

Elevated histamine levels affect digestive, immune and nervous systems. If levels remain high, the adrenalin activation puts the body in a high state of stress which increases stomach acid, disrupts digestion and encourages food sensitivity and microbial infections.

PYROLURIA (urine)

This test measures the levels of 'pyrroles' in the urine. 'Pyroluria' is a biochemical syndrome which is called 'the mauve factor'. The connection in suggesting this test, is the fact that it indicates whether vitamin B6 binds well with zinc. B6 is the co-factor of zinc, without this combined function zinc is unable to do its job well in the body. Zinc and vitamin B6 are depleted by the binding effect of pyrroles.

The 'mauve factor' (termed Kryptopyrrole) in urine, indicates poor binding ability of vitamin B6 and zinc. Clinical signs of this disorder include, nausea, white spots on the fingernails, a sweetish breath odour and occasional abdominal pain in the upper left quadrant. There may also be stretch marks on the skin (white lines on breasts, stomach or any area of expansion), sensitivity to sunlight and tremors or spasms.

Testing to see if vitamin B6 and zinc are biochemically active may be considered in cases of poor digestion, chronic stress, poor blood sugar balance or hormonal disturbances.

THINK ZINC

Another effect of stress is that it reduces not only zinc levels which together with vitamin B6 are needed for producing stomach acid, balancing blood sugar and reproductive hormone production, but also vitamin C and B vitamins. Zinc is in fact required for hundreds of biochemical body functions and many enzyme reactions in the body.

COMPREHENSIVE ADRENAL STRESS PROFILE (saliva)

Measures adrenal hormones, cortisol, DHEA, and secretory IgA.

Researchers investigated the negative impact of stress on the immune system and the Autonomic Nervous System, showing that stress is implicated in inflammatory bowel disease (IBD) and an 'overload' of psychological stress is associated with irritable bowel syndrome (IBS). They also stated that "As many as one in three individuals suffer from stress and some sort of allergic disorder", with an increased prevalence in all countries world-wide.[8]

SIBO BREATH TEST (small intestinal bacterial overgrowth)

This test measures hydrogen and methane gases in the breath, after an oral dose of a sugar solution containing lactulose and glucose.

A test to consider: for IBS, abdominal pain linked to sugar consumption, diarrhoea, steatorrhea (fatty stools), cramping, gas bloating, foul smelling stools.

Eating a carbohydrate rich meal and certainly sugar, can set off symptoms within an hour of eating. Overconsumption of carbohydrates and inadequate digestion over time, can result in bacterial overgrowth.

Bacterial overgrowth of the small intestine can often mimic other digestive disorders, so this test can distinguish the difference and can accurately diagnose carbohydrate intolerance.

Hydrogen is only produced by bacteria in the process of breaking down carbohydrates.

Typical fasting breath samples contain less than 10ppm of breath hydrogen or methane. A level seen on a test result of greater than 20ppm, show evidence of bacterial overgrowth.

COELIAC AND GLUTEN SENSITIVITY (blood test)

A test for suspected sensitivity to gluten in grains.

To be considered for: IBS, Crohn's disease, colitis, diverticulitis, chronic diarrhoea, gastric ulceration, abdominal cramps, foul smelling stools, food sensitivity. Coeliac disease develops from an intolerance to gluten. This disorder is covered in the next chapter.

LACTOSE INTOLERANCE BREATH TEST

To be considered where dairy intolerance is evident, bearing in mind that one can also react to the casein (protein) content in milk, and dairy being a primary source of intolerance can also be triggered by a wheat allergy or vice versa. A test should be considered if sensitivity still exists on re-introduction of dairy after an elimination diet.

This test measures hydrogen levels in breath, following a lactose oral drink.

Lactose is the milk sugar found in dairy. Lactase is the digestive enzyme that breaks it down. Human levels of lactase vary across races. In South East Asia, there is almost a 100% deficiency of this enzyme, with southern Italy and Turkey close behind. North west Europeans and Scandinavians have a level of 3–8% deficiency.[9]

TOXIC ELEMENT CLEARANCE TEST (urine test)
Measures urinary excretion of toxic elements from industry, medical, environmental sources, that may be displacing nutrients in the cell, compromising digestion and undermining health throughout the body. Important assessment of liver function and detoxification processes.

VITAMIN PROFILE (blood serum test)
Measures an array of vitamins, and red blood cell magnesium, if required.

HAIR MINERAL ANALYSIS (hair sample)
Measures mineral elements and toxic elements present in cell structures.

Mineral content of hair mimics the mineral content of your tissues; minerals are involved in all enzyme reactions in the body and are vital for digestion. Vitamins and minerals work synergistically in the body.

There are many reasons for deficiency – poor digestion, absorption, stress, improper dietary balance, inherited deficiencies and heavy metal toxicity, such as lead, arsenic, mercury, cadmium, aluminium, antimony, all of which can displace minerals in the cells.

Metabolic dysfunction, slow or fast metabolism, toxic metals/mineral ratio and significant mineral ratios are shown.

For instance, the zinc/copper, the calcium/magnesium and sodium/potassium ratios, should be in a good reference range for digestion to be optimal.

FOOD INTOLERANCE AND SENSITIVITY TESTS:

ANTIBODIES

Different antibodies are produced in the blood by the immune system in response to antigens (foods, microbes or other substances that provoke an immune reaction).

Antibodies are highly specialised protein molecules that defend and protect your body against attack, they can recognise foreign matter, and aid the immune cells in fighting invasion of damaging bugs, toxins and any food material that the body feels poses a threat.

In the case of food sensitivity, it may not always be the case that the food item in its natural form is antigenic (causing the reaction).

The body can become sensitive and intolerant to the manner of manufacture; herbicides, pesticides, gene alteration, chemical manipulation, food chemical additives, colourings, preservatives, and all the unnatural practices that the food had been exposed to, before and after harvest.

Antibodies are divided into five categories called Immunoglobulins:

- **IgA** – prevents colonisation by pathogens, and resides in mucosal areas, the gut, the respiratory tract, the urogenital tract
- **IgG** – is responsible for the delayed food sensitivity reactions. It does not activate the defensive proteins in the blood, called the complement system, the proteins that cause inflammation
- **IgE** – binds to allergens (a type of antigen that produces vigorous response) and produces allergies rather than food sensitivities. These reactions can be life threatening, with the onset of anaphylactic shock. The IgE attaches itself to mast cells which are distributed throughout the body. When

provoked by an antigen the mast cell releases histamine a hormone that causes redness and inflammation, blood vessels become dilated and muscles contract and degradation of threatening microbes takes place. This antibody is designed to protect against parasites but is so sensitive, food antigens can set off a cascade of reactions. The antibody is responsible for all the allergic reactions, hives, rashes, itching

- **IgD** – aids the immune system and supports its function to produce antimicrobial factors
- **IgM** – eliminates pathogens in the early stage of invasion, before the IgG antibody moves into action

IgG FOOD ANTIBODY ASSESSMENT (blood serum test)
Assesses both IgE and IgG antibodies.

This test is suitable for both immediate allergic reactions and delayed food sensitivities.

ALLERGIX test for IgG – available as a blood finger-prick test and full blood serum

CYREX TESTS (blood serum) – five panels for antibody assessment of gastrointestinal disorders:

- Intestinal-antigenic permeability screen
- Wheat/gluten proteome reactivity and autoimmunity
- Gluten – associated cross-reactive foods and food sensitivity
- Multiple food immune reactivity screen
- Irritable bowel/sibo screen

This is just a guide to the many laboratory tests available to assess gastrointestinal function. A Functional Medicine or Nutritional Therapist practitioner will provide a guided choice of appropriate tests in relation to your presenting symptoms and medical history.

A SAMPLE RESULT:
COMPREHENSIVE DIGESTIVE STOOL ANALYSIS

Digestion	Chymotrypsin normal, putrefactive short chain fatty acids within reference range. Meat fibres outside range. **Recommend Betaine Hydrochloride (HCL), and protease protein digesting enzymes**
Absorption	Long chain fatty acids and faecal fat elevated out of reference range. **Recommend lipase, fat splitting pancreatic enzyme, lecithin, bile salts and botanical support for bile acid production to aid absorption, taurine and Betaine HCL. magnesium, biotin and vitamins B 1,2,5 to aid fat digestion/absorption**
Metabolic Markers	pH 5.9 (ideal range 6.1–7.9). **Recommend avoid all sugar, alcohol, take Betaine HCL and broad based pancreatic enzymes. Suspect SIBO**
Short chain fatty acid distribution	Acetate out of reference range. **Recommend Betaine HCL, pancreatic enzymes, digestive herbs, increase fibre in diet, multi nutrients + Essential fatty acids. Suspect SIBO** Propionate under reference range and **undetected. Recommend increase soluble fibre and water, probiotics, fructo-oligosaccharides (FOS) and inulin prebiotics**
Immunology	Faecal Lactoferrin positive; implies active inflammation present. **Recommend antimicrobial treatment and anti-inflammatory diet**

Macroscopic	Normal colour, normal mucus, occult blood positive. **Recommend ruling out iron deficiency anaemia (refer to GP) for assessment**
Beneficial bacteria	Lactobacillus species 2+ (ideal range 4+). **Recommend Lactobacillus acidophilus and broad-spectrum probiotics.** Bifidobacterium 2+ (ideal range 4+). **Recommend Bifidobacterium and broad-spectrum probiotics.** Escherichia coli 4+ within ideal range
Additional bacteria	Non-pathogenic Haemolytic escherichia coli 2+. **No action**
Mycology	Candida albicans 2+. **Recommend anti-candida diet, sugar and yeast-free, berberine, caprylic acid, garlic, uva ursi, undecyclenic acid**
Parasitology	Blastocystis hominis many. **Recommend botanical anti-parasitic treatment – berberine, artemisia, uva ursi** Dientamoeba fragilis few. Requires the same as above White blood cells rare. **Recommend immune support supplementation**

FOR ALL TESTING PROCEDURES, IT IS HIGHLY ADVISABLE TO CONSULT AN APPROPRIATELY TRAINED PRACTITIONER. FOR ANALYSIS, ADVICE AND TREATMENT RECOMMENDATIONS

Practitioners use their own choice of laboratories. There are many digestive function tests available online but without expert advice for analysis, it could be money ill-spent and present a potential damaging risk to health to self-medicate without expert monitering.

The immune system protects your body against invasion by foreign bodies – microbial organisms and their toxic products. The efficiency of your own immune system function is greatly influenced by your genetic make-up, as well as environmental factors, diet, lifestyle and stress. Immune function can also be undermined by damaging effects of pathogenic organisms in the gut.

One study concluded "The immune system itself, can also suffer pathological consequences because allergies, inflammatory tissue damage and autoimmune diseases can result from the ongoing battle between the immune system and an invading agent."[10]

PARASITES

It is mistakenly thought that parasite infection only occurs in tropical areas, and whilst it is true there is a higher prevalence in these parts, it also holds true that infection is wide spread throughout other areas of the world which have more temperate climates. Parasites live off the host (and thrive on sugar), and in doing so can cause untold damage in the gut or systemically in any part of the body. They are multi-celled organisms, that depend on the food you eat for sustenance.

It had been estimated in 1986 that over 30% of the world's population were infested with parasites, and the figures were rising annually.[11]

Figures today represent much higher levels and judging by positive parasite test results seen over many years in my practice, this indicates a failure of the natural defence mechanisms and lowered immune response in individuals.

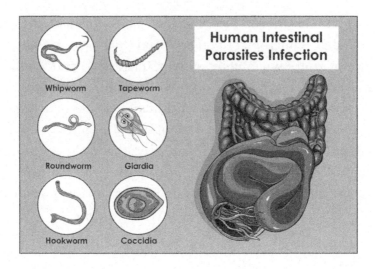

SYMPTOMS include:

Nausea, flatulence, gastric pain and tenderness, backache, joint or muscle pain, abdominal cramps, diarrhoea, food intolerance, weight loss, chronic fatigue, constipation, dizziness and allergic reactions. IBS, itchy ears or on other areas on the body, being more hungry than normal. Eating well but losing weight. General nervous or grumpy disposition, skin conditions, insomnia, tooth grinding, blurry vision or forgetfulness. Stools that may contain some blood and excess mucus.

There are many varieties of parasites including pinworms, round worms and tape worms. Thorough cleansing and purging of the bowels is necessary, combined with comprehensive immune support and a sugar-free diet.

Eradication can be achieved with strong medication, but invariably with some degree of disruption in the balance of healthy organisms in the gut plus the risk of possible damage to the epithelial lining.

Potent botanical agents are highly successful in eradicating parasites without any untoward side-effects. Artemisia annua – a powerful herb has even been shown to eradicate malaria, far more efficiently than anti-malarial drugs.[12] Wild crafted oregano oil has been mentioned as being very effective against parasites in medical studies: www.zanehellas.com

VIRUSES

These organisms do not live off the host but are self-limiting by the action of the host defences, your immune system. They are microscopic pathogens that do not replicate, do not have a cell structure and seize energy from host cells, to infect living cells and tissues in the body.

SYMPTOMS include:

Fever, inflammation, muscle and joint aches, pains, low immunity. Infection can be of acute or chronic nature. Sometimes viruses can become latent which can cause life-long persistent infections. The virus is present but only gets activated when a person is under extreme stress or is suffering from other microbial infections.

Antibiotic treatment has absolutely no effect on viral infection. Antiviral medication can be harsh on the system and disrupt the gut microbiome.

Again, botanical treatment is highly successful and works relatively quickly with no side-effects. I have seen improvement within an hour or two in acute attacks.

BACTERIA

Are living organisms larger than viruses. They live just about everywhere, but within humans, they have ability to multiply rapidly, given certain conditions that favour overgrowth. Pathogenic, unfriendly bacteria live together with friendly, beneficial bacteria in the gut; this is perfectly normal, providing their levels are kept under control with a healthy lifestyle and good dietary habits.

Humans have a very diverse microbial flora, that is easily disturbed by a faulty diet and lifestyle or prolonged stress. Healthy bacteria produce B vitamins and vitamin K in the gut, deter invaders, protect the host from toxins, regulate cholesterol and help stimulate peristalsis which can physically aid the removal of toxins and pathogenic material.

Non-beneficial putrefactive bacteria called Bacteroides, are responsible for decaying matter in the large bowel. They favour a diet of fat and protein, which increases their output of undesirable metabolites. These include such substances as urea, ammonia, phenols, all of which can contribute to many disease patterns, particularly with degenerative disease, such as arthritis, neurological diseases, cardiovascular disease and cancer.

SIGNS OF BACTERIAL INFECTION:

Odorous flatulence, IBS, stomach cramps, fever and chills, digestive problems, food sensitivities, diarrhoea, constipation, stomach pains, urinary tract infections, poor wound healing, respiratory tract infections, sexually transmitted disease, skin infections, food poisoning.

By improving the gut environment, taking probiotic treatment, and using natural antibacterial botanicals, eradication and healthy balance can be restored.

YEAST INFESTATION

Yeasts resemble parasites and live on the lining of the gut wall, and on any mucosal surface in the body. If the gut and digestive system remains healthy, there is little likelihood of fungal overgrowth as the organisms are opportunistic and will flourish in certain environments. The following circumstances can promote fungal overgrowth, it can be localised or in a mycelial form – becoming systemic and travelling to any part of the body.

COMMON CAUSES OF FUNGAL OVERGROWTH:

- The contraceptive pill and HRT

- Regular intake of alcohol which feeds yeasts
- Living in damp mouldy conditions
- Overuse of antibiotics and other drugs
- Over consumption of sugar, bread and yeasted products

SYMPTOMS OF FUNGAL OVERGROWTH:

IBS, abdominal pain, bloating, flatulence, heart-burn, loose stools, indigestion, anal itching, fatigue, stiffness and aching all over, food sensitivity and cravings for sugar, fuzzy head-headedness, poor concentration, brain fog, blurred vision, chemical sensitivity to fumes and perfumes, athletes foot, recurrent thrush, cystitis and fungal skin disorders.

Anti-fungal botanical treatment combined with intense targeted anti-fungal dietary strategies, and long-term recommendations for maintenance, will result in successful eradication of fungal overgrowth.

PART II

CASE HISTORIES FROM CLINICAL PRACTICE

Real names have been changed to protect the identity of the individual.

CASE HISTORY ONE

SUSAN consulted me with symptoms of IBS, that had been ongoing intermittently two or three times yearly for twenty years. The symptoms had recently increased in frequency, with three episodes occurring in the last month. There was also a question of whether she suffered with candida fungal overgrowth, as symptoms improved when sugar, wine and yeast were avoided, and stress levels reduced.

MEDICAL HISTORY:

Susan had undergone surgery; an appendectomy and tonsillectomy at twenty years of age, and a partial removal of her thyroid gland a few years later. She had used acupuncture for two to three months post surgically and was not currently on permanent medication. Antacid medication was being taken as and when the need arose. HRT had been prescribed in the past for a short period but then discontinued.

Her father had suffered with asthma and emphysema, and her mother had developed late onset diabetes. An aunt had suffered ovarian cancer. There was a family history of allergies.

Three years previously Susan had suffered with ME for a period of nine months, following exposure to Tamiflu.

She suffered dry skin, with menopause onset eight years previously, which had been alleviated with soya supplements and cream.

Twelve years ago, whilst abroad, Susan had suffered with amoebic dysentery, probably, she felt, due to swallowing swimming pool water. This was treated with anti-parasitic treatment. She had also picked up ringworm prior to the dysentery episode.

She had spent three years in India on a vegetarian diet, which she felt at the time suited her.

She had an allergy to penicillin, experiencing body rash and mouth ulcers with exposure.

CLINICAL OBSERVATIONS:

Cramps and tenderness in the stomach, stomach pains, flatulence, bloating with distension. No diarrhoea but loose stools and irritable bowel. She experienced indigestion on a regular basis, with frequent stomach upsets. In the last six months, she had experienced weight loss of half a stone and was currently eight stone two pounds. Her normal weight was between eight and a half to nine stone.

Susan was worried about the weight loss, and had difficulty putting on weight. Her skin was very dry. She appeared to be under a degree of stress, had a poor tolerance to pain, worked long hours, multi-tasked and was a very 'driven' type of individual. Having a good sleep pattern, Susan was a 'morning' person who needed to sleep over eight hours. She did regular exercise, yoga, swimming, walking, considered herself fit, though having energy slumps around three in the afternoon.

Wine, sugar and yeast caused bouts of digestive discomfort. Appetite was good, despite feeling many foods did not agree with her. She lived on a busy road, close to an agricultural area.

CURRENT DIET:

Susan admitted to not chewing food well, drank unfiltered tap water and regularly ate her meals under stressful conditions. Meat was eaten more than once daily, often with browned and barbecued food. Food was also fried at elevated temperatures in oils, which produced undesirable smoke toxins. Plastic and aluminium foil was used for food wrapping.

- Alcohol intake was low, one glass of whisky per week. Oily fish was eaten more than three times weekly. Yoghurt was eaten daily, she generally avoided sugar and salt. 50% of the diet was raw fruit and vegetables
- Normal diet included white flour processed grains and non-organic products. Fruit and vegetables were not washed before eating. Chocolate and coffee was avoided. Favourite foods were mixed roasted nuts, vegetables, pulses, humus and fruit
- Breakfast consisted of porridge with honey weekdays and cooked meals with rye bread and eggs at weekends. Jasmine tea was consumed daily. Lunch and dinners contained adequate variety of vegetables, and protein

ASSESSMENT:

Suspected gut microbial infection, possibly parasite and fungal problems. Dysbiosis. Poor digestion and absorption – stress related. Nutrient deficiencies and poor dietary choices. Blood sugar imbalance. Low stomach acid.

TREATMENT RECOMMENDATIONS

DIET:

Recommended avoiding all sugar (including honey), yeast, fermented foods, alcohol, red meat and pork, wheat and dairy (excluding yoghurt and butter for probiotics and butyric acid which is beneficial for the gut).

To reduce fruit high in sugar and starchy foods bananas and potatoes but to increase leafy dark green vegetables. To eat light proteins – white fish (no seafood), well cooked chicken, lamb and eggs. To use wheat-free wholegrains, such as gram flour, buckwheat and rice flour and to continue with rye or spelt (old variety of wheat with a different structure to modern wheat).

I did not suspect gluten to be an issue. Considering parasites, I advised continuing with jasmine tea as this has anti-microbial effects, as well as culinary herbs, garlic and sweet spices. Other recommendations included – avoiding dietary practices such as frying in very high temperature, which produces burnt, overly browned meats; this can be carcinogenic and is not recommended. Avoiding plastic wrapping where possible; chemicals in plastic can migrate into food and act as hormone disrupters. Likewise, aluminium foil as this can react with acid foods and release toxic aluminium into the body.

To apply stress-free eating conditions, chew well and take time to digest. Drink filtered or bottled water to regularly hydrate, avoiding tap water, which is often full of undesirable chemicals and heavy metals, even though it is clean from a microbial viewpoint.

Eating unroasted nuts would be more nutritious, the roasting process damages sensitive essential fats.

INITIAL SUPPLEMENT PROGRAMME FOR ONE MONTH:

(Only to be started after the stool test had been completed)

This strategy allows earlier relief from symptoms, the programme was adjusted when test results were to hand.

- A multi vitamin and mineral formula with high dose B vitamins, 1 with breakfast
- Berberine and grapefruit seed botanical anti-microbial formula, with gentian root, golden seal, artemisia, quassia bark, black walnut hull and garlic, 2 at bedtime on an empty stomach

(This product is most effective in dealing with parasites, fungi, viruses and bacteria)

- Broad-spectrum digestive enzymes, 1 before each meal
- Artichoke plus complex, with milk thistle, artichoke leaf, dandelion, and fringe tree. 1 at midday meal and evening meal. Caution drug interation
- Multi strain advanced probiotic, 1 with breakfast

We had telephone contact for advice on loose stools, cramping and bloating (normal whilst eliminating parasites). I recommended pectin powder, a high potency digestive aid with Betaine hydrochloride and specific enzymes, plus slippery elm with marshmallow and gamma oryzanol from rice, all of which soothe the intestinal tract, and help to buffer the mucosal lining from irritation from food. Susan questioned whether she was tolerating the artichoke supplement. She felt it did not agree with her, so reducing adjustments were made. Fennel tea was added.

BIOCHEMICAL TESTS RECOMMENDED:
Comprehensive Digestive Stool Analysis with Parasitology

RESULTS:

- Adequate protein digestion

- Long chain fatty acids, cholesterol, and total faecal fat were elevated out of the reference range (fat loss in the stools)
- Phospholipids and triglycerides were normal
- (This suggested fat malabsorption with possible bile salt and pancreatic insufficiency)
- Acetate, one of the short chain fatty acids was out of the reference range, suggesting dysbiosis, an imbalance in bowel ecology (SCFAs are the end products of bacterial fermentation of dietary fibre)
- Beneficial bacteria, both Lactobacillus and Bifidobacterium species were below optimal levels at 2+ respectively
- Faecal Lactoferrin was positive, an inflammatory marker, indicating an active inflammatory process
- Occult blood was negative
- Parasites, the results showed positive for Blastocystis Hominis
- Rare yeasts observed microscopically

SECOND SUPPLEMENT PROGRAMME FOR THREE MONTHS:

The first programme was amended to include 1 slippery elm capsule, 20 mins before each meal.

- 1 high potency digestive aid with Betaine Hydrochloride/ Pepsin before main meal in the evening
- A multi digestive enzyme formula, 1 before each of the other two meals
- Continuing with the rest of the previously recommended programme
- Reducing the artichoke dose to 1 daily main meal and gradually build up to 3 daily again to achieve a better tolerance

There were many emails over the next weeks to clarify the new supplement programme, as Susan travelled a lot and needed assurance that she was taking it in accordance with my instructions. This was outlined in a precise chart and her confidence was reassured, when I emphasised that the effects she was experiencing from the treatment, were normal and to be expected. And if in doubt whilst traveling – I recommended discontinuing all supplements until we could make contact.

Susan occasionally did not feel like eating when her stomach was unsettled. I advised her to avoid supplements when active inflammation was occurring and eat a bland diet with light protein, well cooked – chicken, fish, eggs, no salad and lightly cooked vegetables including root vegetables, avoiding extra stress on the digestive system.

Susan queried whether she should be gluten free as well, I did not feel this was appropriate and that the wheat itself, which can be pro-inflammatory, was most likely the problem food.

Her blood sugar levels kept fluctuating with such an inconsistent eating pattern.

I emphasised the need to hydrate with plain quality water. To store glucose from carbohydrate foods – the body needs water – 1 molecule of glucose needs 2 molecules of water. and having protein at each carbohydrate meal also balances blood sugar levels by the action of slowing digestive processes and promoting efficient storage of glucose reserves in muscles and liver.

To ensure all grains were wholegrains as nutrient dense complex carbohydrate, taking 2–3 hours to be digested, as opposed to white processed flours that give a quick sugar fix.

These measures help blood sugar balance and stop sugar cravings. Gradually the eating pattern improved, but she still experienced fluctuating appetite swings. I encouraged her to eat regularly regardless of appetite, to maintain a healthy weight.

The artichoke supplement was not proving compatible, so it was put aside and added in again a few days later, after the gut had settled down again.

Susan had a long trip abroad planned. I double checked her supplement chart and ensured she was happy with the programme before she went. On arriving after a long flight, she again experienced very loose stools. I suggested 500–1000mg of calcium citrate daily to help slow the transit time and firm up the stools, but only as an emergency treatment, short-term, to make her more comfortable on holiday, as alkalising calcium in the gut whilst on anti-microbial treatment, is counter-productive. Apples, bananas and pectin powder were also recommended to help firm stools.

Within three weeks, Susan was feeling comfortable and symptom-free, with only slight loose stools which were alleviated by the apples and bananas and the citrus pectin powder. The calcium was then discontinued.

RESULTS OF SECOND FOLLOW-UP ASSESSMENT:

- Pectin powder had helped to firm up stools
- Gut problems now under control, no stomach or gut pains.
- Felt energetic and slept well
- Transit time still a little fast, with frequent stools plus frequent urination (I explained that this was normal whilst on anti-microbial therapy, as the body was eliminating destroyed parasites and toxins)
- Weight loss was still occurring and Susan had now lost one and a half stone in total (Parasites feed off the host and are notorious for causing weight loss)

RE-TESTED WITH CDSA/P

RESULTS:
- Normal absorption of long chain fatty acids, now within the reference range, suggesting normal fat absorption
- Short chain fatty acid distribution, now all within the reference range, suggesting an improved balance of beneficial bacteria in the gut

- Lactoferrin, still positive, indicating active inflammation
- Occult blood, positive (recommended GP assessment)
- Beneficial bacteria, Lactobacillus species and Bifidobacterium levels improved to 3+ and 4+
- Campylobacter antigen marker was positive, indicating the presence of pathogenic bacteria of the bacillus species, which can cause bacterial diarrhoea, with or without the presence of blood (Often once anti-microbial treatment is initiated, new species of pathogens can emerge and be detected in the stool, indicating the complexity of the gut microbiome)
- Parasites, still evident, Blastocystis Hominis at moderate levels
- White blood cells, rare, indicating the immune system has been activated to defend the body from attack by pathogenic bacteria

NEXT ASSESSMENT:

Susan's weight was seven and a half stone but had now stabilised.

She had referred to her GP for a colonoscopy, which showed no evidence of any serious condition, inflammation, however was noted. Prior to the appointment, I asked her to mention the positive Campylobacter specific antigen result. No action was taken.

Her diet was adjusted to address the weight loss, increasing breakfast calorie intake, a cooked breakfast of eggs on rye bread, porridge or sugar-free muesli, bananas, apple and nuts. The bananas although a source of starch and sugar, provided comfort in reducing the rapid transit time. No other fruit was taken.

She ate feta cheese and had no ill effects, salmon, meat stock soup, rice, avocado and quinoa, green vegetables, salad and potatoes; not an ideal food from a starch point of view (sugar that feeds microbes) but a food she felt helped ease her fluctuating blood sugar levels and calmed her gut. This shows the varied diet strategies required for individual treatment plans.

Full fat yoghurt in the diet added healthy bacteria and provided fat and protein, and an increased intake of calories throughout the day, helped to stop the rapid weight loss. Goats and sheep cheese had been introduced. Nuts, were beginning to cause gut problems, I asked her to avoid them, whilst on other high fat foods, as the body was probably having difficulty metabolising the increased level of fats.

Emphasis was put on bitter teas to aid bile and liver function and supply anti-microbial support, chicory, dandelion root tea, ginger. Yogi teas with spice and black pepper, but only if tolerated, olive leaf tea, peppermint, thyme, oregano, and chamomile (for a soothing effect). To increase garlic and onions for a source of sulphur which helps detoxification.

THIRD SUPPLEMENT PROGRAMME FOR THREE MONTHS:

The focus was on liver support and conjugating (binding) botanical agents for improving detoxification pathways. Once parasites and unhealthy bacteria are killed off, they need excreting; this job is done by the liver and is fully explained in chapter 7.

- Multi Liver Formula, contains specific amino acids, known to be necessary for the conjugation of pathogens and toxins prior to excretion, 1 between meals three times daily
- Milk Thistle Complex, 15 drops twice daily in water between meals
- Microflora Guard, botanical oils and probiotics, 1 daily with main meal
- Berberine and Oregano Complex (a formula designed for a range of undesirable organisms), 2 daily on empty stomach (early a.m. and bedtime)
- Artichoke Plus, 1 daily main meal
- A high strength probiotic, 1 with breakfast

FINAL TELEPHONE CONSULTATION ASSESSMENT:

Susan had felt well for the last 3 months, and free of all symptoms. All supplements had been well tolerated and she felt fine on the programme. Unfortunately, more travel abroad, with a change in diet, had prompted another bout of cramping and bloating. She had eaten a lot of cheese as dietary choice was limited. Weight remained the same, with no increase, and her appetite had diminished, until the gut problem had settled.

She had been trying to increase calorie intake, with extra cheese, despite the appetite loss.

ADJUSTED SUPPLEMENT PROGRAMME FOR ONE MONTH:

- High dose digestive enzymes, 1 with main meal
- Betaine HCL, 1 with every protein meal
- Berberine at bedtime, 2 on an empty stomach
- Multi vitamin and mineral formula with high dose B vitamins, 1 at breakfast
- A high strength lactobacillus acidophilus probiotic, 1 daily with any meal
- Lipase a fat-splitting digestive enzyme, 1 daily with main meal
- Magnesium Taurate, 1 daily with main meal, to provide support for fat digestion

FURTHER TESTS ORDERED:

FOOD INTOLERANCE

This test could have been run earlier but the practicality of treating both microbial issues and severe weight loss in an individual constantly travelling, with a potential limited diet, had to be weighed up with the initial presenting health problems. It was now appropriate to know which foods had to be avoided on a long-term basis.

RESULTS:

Showed an intolerance to cow's milk but not to other processed dairy products. Intolerance to mixed nuts and egg white was indicated but at low levels. This suggested secondary intolerance.

FINAL RECOMMENDATIONS GIVEN

DIET:

Nuts, egg white, and all dairy were removed from the diet. Sugar and wheat avoidance was important to maintain future health.

CDSA/P SECOND RE-TEST

FINAL RESULTS:
- Digestion – markers normal
- Absorption – markers normal
- All Metabolic – markers normal
- Lactoferrin – negative
- Occult blood – negative
- Pathogenic bacteria – negative
- Parasites – negative
- Low Lactobacillus species

An excellent outcome, apart from low levels again of healthy Lactobacillus species. This indicated a need for more lactic acid products in the diet and focus on healthy fibre balance.

On discharge, I recommended one quality multi-nutrient formula daily at breakfast for long-term maintenance of health, a month's treatment with a Lactobacillus probiotic and dietary advice to improve stomach acid and digestion for long-term maintenance of gastrointestinal health.

Susan has kept very well to date, with no gut problems, reaching her ideal weight and enjoying most foods including dates, figs and even dried fruit and yeasted products, dairy, nuts in moderation and occasional alcohol. She continues to avoid wheat and sugar.

CASE HISTORY TWO

LUCY consulted me with severe allergy to all fish and shellfish. Candida fungal overgrowth, severe lactose intolerance, wheat intolerance, low energy and poor digestion.

MEDICAL HISTORY:

- At age 5, suffered with recurring bouts of tonsillitis and was given regular doses of antibiotics in childhood
- Endometriosis diagnosed at age 25 and problems with infertility around this time. Still currently seeking natural fertility support
- Family history of allergies
- Anaphylactic shock to fish (tuna) as a young adult
- Family history of heart disease

CLINICAL OBSERVATION:

Currently suffered with low energy, far less than it used to be, but exercised regularly and felt fit. Until 2 years ago, was highly active with horse riding.

Suffered with PMS – irritability and depression, chronic thrush with vaginal itching and cystitis. Periods were regular, she did not use contraception. Lucy found Agnus castus a herbal product proved beneficial for the hormonal imbalance but zinc supplementation caused an increase in symptoms. Endometriosis less problematic than 10 years previous. Was breast-fed.

Suffered with flatulence, bloating and anal irritation. She had problems with food sensitivity and allergy problems. Food intolerance, stool and saliva tests were run in the past year.

She was tested positive for fish allergy and had bacterial and fungal overgrowth. Anti-microbial herbal treatment had been carefully followed, but she was still suffering with gut problems and frequent sore throats.

Dairy caused gut cramps, odorous flatulence and diarrhoea, so had been avoided.

Slept over 8 hours, was a morning person and had a poor tolerance to pain.

Spent a good deal of time on computer.

Had many mercury fillings.

Worked very hard, multi tasked and had a persistent need for achievement.

Impatience with people and situations that hindered progress.

CURRENT DIET:

- Wheat and dairy free for 8 years. Drinks soya milk in place of dairy
- Eats sugar and chocolate regularly, enjoys Earl Grey tea – 5 cups daily
- Low alcohol intake, as tends to have insomnia with increased intake, finds the herb milk thistle helps
- Does not chew food well, but has a good appetite, and takes time to eat and digest under restful conditions
- Avoids additives in food, drinks filtered or bottled water
- Takes only 7 portions of raw fruit/vegetables weekly, does not wash produce before eating
- Eats processed white rice
- Breakfast consists of fruit smoothie and 2 oat crackers, honey, soya milk and Earl Grey tea

ASSESSMENT:

Suspected hormonal imbalance, adrenal stress, leaky gut, mal-digestion and absorption, mineral deficiencies, possible copper toxicity due to negative reactions to zinc, microbial infection and immune dysfunction. Possible heavy metal toxicity. Poor dietary balance with high carbohydrate and sugar intake and reduced protein and fat.

TREATMENT RECOMMENDATIONS

DIET:

Avoid all sugar, yeast, alcohol, fermented products, follow an anti-candida diet (information on this approach in chapter 5). Dietary hand-out sheets given.

Chew food well, increase intake of fresh vegetables and salad which are well washed, reduce fruit to only berries and tart apples, eat wheat-free wholegrains, but not processed white flour products, which can give a quick 'sugar' fix and upset blood sugar balance.

Avoid all dairy and red meat but increase protein for hormonal balance.

Change breakfast habit.

Avoid fruit smoothies (not appropriate for candida sufferers), honey, soya milk and Earl Grey tea. Recommend wheat and sugar-free muesli for breakfast with coconut or nut milk, added ground almonds and seeds, blueberries and coconut cream, followed by an egg.

Earl Grey tea contains bergamot that can irritate the gut lining, to substitute with other herbal teas of choice or green tea with jasmine.

Avoid chocolate, which has stimulatory affects and contains sugar and all soya products which can negatively affect hormone balance. Replace with sugar-free nut and coconut milks. Coconut contains caprylic acid which has anti-fungal properties, together with olive oil, garlic and onions. Eat linseeds and walnuts for omega 3 and 6 essential fats, until fish intolerance could be assessed.

INITIAL SUPPLEMENT PROGRAMME FOR ONE MONTH:

until tests results were to hand.

- High dose digestive enzymes, 1 with each meal
- Cranberry Plus, (vitamin C, probiotics and cranberry powder), 1 dose daily with breakfast (beneficial for fungal infections)
- Female multiple vitamins and minerals, 1 daily with breakfast
- Magnesium citrate, 2 daily with midday and evening meal
- Continue with Agnus castus and milk thistle

BIOCHEMICAL TESTS:

Hair Mineral Analysis (hair mineral levels reflect body tissue status) and an Adrenal Stress Profile (saliva) was ordered.

RESULTS:

Adrenal fatigue was noted, with the lab comment that abnormalities seen were due to excessive stimulation taken place over time. Cortisol, the stress hormone was outside the reference range on 4 samples taken over a period of 12 hours.

Copper toxicity was seen on the HMA hair test. The zinc/copper ratio was low, indicating low zinc and excess copper. Normally zinc to copper ratio is high not low. Zinc is required for digestive function, hormonal balance and blood sugar stability amongst many other enzyme functions. Copper promotes fungal overgrowth.

It was notable that zinc supplementation caused PMT symptoms to increase. Zinc and copper balance one another, elevated copper would negatively affect the absorption of zinc.

A high calcium/magnesium ratio, indicating magnesium deficiency.

A high sodium/potassium ratio, indicating acute stress or inflammatory processes.

Low hair iron was noted, indicating low tissue reserves.

Elevated aluminium was evident.

SECOND MONTHLY ASSESSMENT:

Lucy commented on the first month's programme, she felt an overall improvement in health. The cranberry had helped the sore throat and she felt her menstrual cycle itself had improved despite an increase in PMT. I suggested to improve hormonal balance, and help reduce stress, she should increase protein intake by having an egg each morning at breakfast. Adding protein to a carbohydrate meal can calm the autonomic nervous system. Keeping well hydrated helps blood sugar balance and reduces sugar cravings.

Lucy was cautioned that certain supplementation can be harmful if pregnancy occurred, she must take appropriate action in this event and discontinue the programme.

SECOND SUPPLEMENT PROGRAMME FOR THREE MONTHS:

The supplement programme was formulated from the Hair Mineral Analysis Laboratory. Re-testing for assessment is run at 3 months. The treatment plan consisted of metabolic, molecular, glandular supplements, with chelated minerals, dietary aids, and probiotics; specifically designed to correct metabolic and biochemical imbalance linked to mineral excesses and deficiencies. It is a complex process to rebalance minerals, the laboratory products are more finely tuned than individual practitioner protocols.

I included Cranberry Plus in the plan, 1 level teaspoon in water before any meal, plus the milk thistle to give extra liver support.

Liquorice powder DGL was also recommended to address adrenal stress and a possible leaky gut.

Gut tests were planned, post the mineral balancing treatment, considering she would have a 'leaky gut' due to the allergies, and all probability, poor liver detoxification function. Another consideration, was the amount of old mercury fillings present in her mouth, with potential risk of leakage through chewing and degradation.

Correcting mineral imbalance helps bind heavy metals in the body. These toxic elements displace minerals in the cells, so need chelating (binding) and excreting. Mineral balancing programmes address this.

Toxic 'burden' in the body can overwhelm liver detoxification pathways, heavy metal toxicity, mainly from mercury in the mouth, which is highly toxic and should not be in anyone's mouth, is quite common in the older generation. It was, and is, still used in childhood vaccinations, although mostly replaced by aluminium, another damaging metal, following numerous legal cases linked to cases of autism. Nowadays the dangers of mercury toxicity are recognised (apart from the NHS in the UK who still use it as a cheap option).

Lucy had planned to replace her fillings, so I referred her to a biological dentist and treatment was due to commence, after the HMA supplement programme was well underway, with the knowledge that at least this would give some support to protecting the body during removal. It was planned to add split cell chlorella and spirulina to aid excretion of heavy metals.

TELEPHONE UPDATE A MONTH LATER:

Lucy was working for twelve hours per day, was very stressed, had a constant sore throat, fluctuating fever and felt extremely fatigued. She had initially felt very well on the starting dose I recommended with the HMA programme, which was one third of the recommendations from the laboratory. Since increasing the programme under my recommendation, she felt very unwell.

I explained smaller doses working with the pace of the body is much more beneficial as biochemical changes taking place can be extreme in some individuals. I recommended reducing the programme back to a third. I discontinued the liquorice, as it appeared to be not well tolerated, and added the following to the existing HMA programme;

- Immune and anti-microbial support, echinacea and black elderberry, 3 daily between meals

- Acidophilus probiotic 1 daily anytime
- Lysine anti-viral amino acid 500mg, 2 tablets daily with main meal (Vitamin C that was needed for lysine to work well, was already in the full programme)
- Garlic was recommended in the diet

Lucy was notified to stop the programme should further symptoms arise, wait 3 days to allow the liver to perform its role in metabolic balancing, then restart the supplements and to stay on the low dose throughout the three months.

The liver needs to work in tune with the gut and so many changes take place when mineral balancing occurs. The liver metabolises all these processes.

HMA programmes initiate what is called re-tracing, taking the body through biochemical stages to correct mineral imbalance. During this process, latent (hidden) viruses and bacteria in the body can become active again. It is essential to reduce copper levels to control fungal overgrowth.

HMA and treatment protocols expose underlying nutrient imbalance, which often gives a clue as to why earlier anti-microbial treatment wasn't successful in clearing infections.

Following an anti-fungal diet, fungi are destroyed and released into the body, they then need excreting via the liver.

The 'Herxheimer' reaction is a normal response to anti-fungal treatment. It does produce some distressing symptoms, but just requires extra support of the liver.

Lucy's frequent sore throat and low-grade fever during the programme could have been linked to re-tracing or the 'Herxheimer' reaction. Fungal infections, once treated can produce health problems as the body needs to deal with what is called 'die off', it is a significant healing process, as yeasts start dying off in large numbers, the trick is to give time for the liver to clear up the debris for excretion. Stopping treatment for a few days, supporting liver pathways nutritionally and drinking plenty of water helps this process.

A further telephone call 2 weeks later, came with news that Lucy felt very unwell, faint, hot, and had a constant sore throat that was nor clearing. I advised stopping the programme for 1–2 weeks, taking only the immune support and milk thistle with plenty of water to clear out the body. She was coming to the end of the HMA programme and had not had a very pleasant time. This however, was an indication of underlying deeply seated imbalance. Ten days later Lucy felt much better and re-started the programme for the last 3 weeks, experiencing no further problems.

OUTCOME:

Finally finishing the supplements. Her excess body heat normalised, the sore-throat had practically cleared. Lucy felt very active and walked, cycled, rode her horse and was working less hours, she felt stress was under control. Her periods were not as long, there was little cramping, and she felt she was making a lot of progress with her health issues.

She had had cravings for fish which she had always loved, and tentatively tried a small amount of fish, with no adverse reaction, so included it into her diet. She also tried a small amount of spelt bread with no adverse reaction, but she planned to avoid all sugar and alcohol. Dairy had been put to the test and there was no negative reaction, so that too had been added into the diet.

All the fillings had safely been extracted and replaced. I advised a heavy metal binding (chelating) supplement programme, to deal with any residue in the body, with glutathione, cilantro, split cell chlorella, MSM and other mercury binding agents.

A FINAL RE-TEST HMA AND CP Comprehensive Parasitology were ordered as Lucy was keen to proceed with nutritional fertility support.

FINAL RESULTS:

HMA – the re-test changes showed successful elimination of copper.

- The calcium/magnesium ratio had improved, indicating improved magnesium absorption
- The sodium/potassium ratio had dropped, indicating a possible stress protection mechanism by the body in response to getting rid of heavy metals. Sea-salt intake daily, was recommended to help in rebalancing the electrolytes, and getting rid of stress
- The calcium/potassium ratio had increased, not uncommon when one is actively eliminating copper. It was recommended to increase potassium-rich foods. Fruit and vegetables
- There were many improvements and ideally the programme should have carried on for a further 3 months. However, due to an overall improvement in symptoms and the fact that she was no longer intolerant to fish and seafood, dairy and wheat, Lucy decided she was happy with the treatment outcome, and she was obviously in an improved state of health
- Recommendations were to continue with all sugar, yeast and alcohol avoidance for the near future

CP – No parasites or bacterial overgrowth were evident, only low level of yeast overgrowth from Candida albicans at 1+. All levels of beneficial bacteria were 4+, which is a very good outcome. Lucy was then discharged.

CASE HISTORY THREE

RICHARD consulted me with IBS and distressing digestive problems of long-standing.

MEDICAL HISTORY:

- Family history of IBS and gastric disorders
- Parents suffered with diabetes and lung disease

- Onset of Richard's gut problems with stomach pain and constipation, followed a holiday abroad fifteen years ago
- GP diagnosed a duodenal ulcer five years ago, (no colonoscopy performed). Richard doubted the diagnosis as a colonoscopy performed four years ago, could find no signs of a healed ulcer

CLINICAL OBSERVATIONS:

- High stress levels at work due to work overload and management responsibilities
- Suffered with IBS, constipation and alternating diarrhoea, nausea and bouts of vomiting, stomach pains and itchy legs, pain under ribs on the left side
- Lack of energy, pale skin and fatigued and anaemic looking
- Possibility of toxic bowel – felt an increase in energy, post barium enema for colonoscopy four years ago. Felt invigorated when not eating and fasting

CURRENT DIET:

- Vegetarian, (no other family members are vegetarian)
- Dairy-free for four years, apart from yoghurt and cottage cheese, which he tolerates well, instantly feeling more energy
- High intake of eggs – feels well on these
- Protein derived from quinoa and grains
- Is very strict and only buys organic produce
- He avoids sugar and all food additives and reads labels
- Drinks include herb tea, and occasional other varieties. Has occasional alcohol

ASSESSMENT:

Possible dysbiosis, toxic bowel, poor liver function due to inadequate protein intake for detoxification. Adrenal stress, nutrient imbalance, maldigestion, malabsorption and iron deficiency. Low stomach acid. Enzyme insufficiency. Gastric inflammation. Protein and fat deficiency. Acid alkaline imbalance from vegetarian diet.

TREATMENT RECOMMENDATIONS

DIET:

- Avoid wheat and dairy (apart from tolerated forms), alcohol and stimulants – chocolate, cocoa, tea or coffee. Herb teas were fine
- Avoid all sugar, reduce fruits, eat only pears, blueberries, raspberries and bananas (potassium rich)
- Avoid rye and spelt
- To increase intake of protein providing foods, pulses, legumes, amino rich quinoa and amaranth, and healthy grains, buckwheat and oats. Cook all breakfast grains in rice or coconut milk, if not having a cooked breakfast, boost fat and protein with ground hemp seeds (high in protein), ground almonds, mixed seeds, coconut and full fat yoghurt
- Increase intake of unrefined rice – wild or other varieties, rice contains gamma oryzanol which has a healing effect in the gut. Eat eggs daily and protein at each meal (eggs, cottage cheese, yoghurt)
- To eat buckwheat pancakes made with eggs for breakfast with allowable fruit, yoghurt, ground almonds and seeds. Suggest carob powder (contains calcium that helps to de-stress) drink made with sugar-free nut or coconut milk, taken at bedtime, and time allowing in the morning, a full cooked breakfast with mushrooms, falafel, eggs and gently fried potatoes
- Increase nuts and seeds in the diet, (essential fatty acids have a healing effect on the gut lining and are anti-inflammatory), ground almonds on breakfast cereal, linseeds, sunflower and pumpkin seeds. Eat avocados daily for more healthy fat intake and to help reduce stress. Use unrefined olive oil, avocado oil, but avoid all other processed cooking oils

- Eat garlic and onions for sulphur intake, to aid gut cleansing. Eat plenty of varied root and dark green leafy vegetables for fibre, pulses and colourful salad, avoiding tomatoes, until digestion improves. Eat potatoes regularly, in any form (potassium containing, which has a soothing effect on the gut)
- Not to re-heat any food to keep bacterial contamination at a minimum

FIRST SUPPLEMENT PROGRAMME FOR ONE MONTH:

- Psyllium husk powder, 1 dose daily after evening meal. As cleansing fibre for bowels
- Gastro Cleanse formula with botanicals, taken three times daily with meals
- Digestive enzymes with gentle low dose Betaine HCL, 1 with main meal
- Zinc and vitamin B6, 1 daily with breakfast. (Nausea is often linked to zinc deficiency)
- Multi vitamin and mineral formula, 1 daily with breakfast

BIOCHEMICAL TESTS
None recommended initially

MONTHLY FOLLOW-UP ASSESSMENT:

- Richard reported a 50% improvement in his IBS and digestive symptoms
- IBS had improved considerably, no nausea or vomiting, stools were regulating in frequency and formation
- Itchy legs had improved, much less of a bother
- After 9 months of pain and soreness under left ribcage, a significant improvement but still slightly sore and not completely cleared
- Bloating after the main meal still occurring

- Had a constant lack of energy however, he cycled regularly in charity rides in the past and would like to be more active. He felt he could sleep all day
- Felt very well on buckwheat pancakes as suggested
- Felt calmer in the gut area, experiencing improved digestion when eating more protein with a cooked breakfast
- Starting to feel yoghurt was not so well tolerated after all

COMMENTS:

Given the physical nature of Richard's workload, I felt his protein requirements were much higher than that provided by his current dietary intake, so he was encouraged to focus on protein at each meal. His energy output depended not only on the intake of energy promoting carbohydrates but efficient energy production in the cells, which in turn depends on good nutrient balance. Protein and fat needs to be in correct ratio to the carbohydrate intake for good digestion, otherwise one can become overly acid or alkaline and digestion will falter.

Richard was effectively running on a carbohydrate dominant diet which was not in tune with his metabolic type.

I classified him as a parasympathetic, metabolic type who needed a 'heavy' diet with more fat and protein. Proteins and fat are needed for the structure of enzymes, hormones and every cell in the body. Improving protein intake would result in helping his body produce energy more efficiently. If cell structure is faulty through lack of building materials, it cannot produce energy efficiently.

Citric acid – containing fruit was recommended at a later stage, when the gut had settled. Non-tart apples were added to the diet for the malic acid which helps mineral transport into cells and as an aid to help settle the stomach.

Richard was asked to stop eating yoghurt, as it was obvious from our conversation that the lactic acid in the product was causing localised gastric acidity. Instead crème fraiche was suggested, and later a recommendation to try goat's yoghurt. The protein content is lower than cow's yoghurt, but more easily digested.

Betaine HCL and digestive enzymes, despite being contra-indicated for many gastrointestinal diseases, are often required for dealing with gastrointestinal complaints.

Sometimes the condition has developed initially as an effect of low stomach acid and pancreatic enzyme production, in which case, I have found by starting with a low dose and building up the potency, a good outcome can be achieved.

There are occasions where digestive enzymes and HCL should never be used however, if bleeding is evident and a high degree of inflammation. Once this has cleared, they can be introduced gradually.

SECOND SUPPLEMENT PROGRAMME FOR ONE MONTH:

- Protein powder, 1–2 scoops daily with meals
- Mastik gum capsules for gastric pain, 2 to be taken at bedtime
- Multi vitamin mineral formula with high dose B Vitamins, 2 with breakfast in middle of the meal to avoid gut irritation
- Zinc and vitamin B6, 1 daily main meal of the day
- HCL and pepsin, 1 in the middle of main meal of the day (not to irritate the gut lining)
- Broad spectrum digestive enzymes, 1 daily to start in middle of midday meal, increasing to 1 at breakfast and 1 midday meals
- White willow complex, anti-inflammatory botanical, 1 mid-morning, 1 mid-afternoon

MONTHLY FOLLOW-UP VISIT:

- Progress continues, Richard felt even better this month
- On residual gastric soreness and discomfort, again, Richard felt a 50% improvement and the itchiness on legs was clearing
- Stools had normalised, no diarrhoea or constipation, stools

were also well-formed
- He felt much more energetic and in good health with the extra protein in the diet
- He now ate 2 eggs, olive oil and cottage cheese daily. Richard felt the lactic acid in yoghurt upset him, so would avoid this for the moment. (Not everyone does well on fermented foods regardless of the potential health benefits; this was an example of individuality in dietary requirements.) He enjoyed crème fraiche, so had introduced all other dairy forms, to keep his protein levels high, he also ate pulses on a regular basis
- The only time he felt unwell in the gut was when he was obliged to eat out at work and was forced to eat refined carbohydrates or drink some alcohol

RECOMMENDED THE SAME SUPPLEMENT PROGRAMME FOR ONE MONTH

MONTHLY FOLLOW-UP VISIT:
- Remained very well again on the same programme
- Had no gastric pain or sign of bowel problems
- Had high energy and had started mountain biking and other sports
- Had introduced rye, spelt bread and goat's milk products with goat's yoghurt into the diet, without any problems

RECOMMENDED FOR MAINTENANCE:
- A multi vitamin and mineral formula to be taken with breakfast
Richard was then discharged.

POSTSCRIPT TO THIS CASE

Six months later Richard again consulted me with some gastric pain, though only slight, otherwise he still felt well with high energy.

He had been on holiday, eaten a lot of wheat and drank alcohol as he felt he was cured, and the pain had returned. He also felt a bit 'foggy-headed' as he described it.

The mastik gum helped again to ease the discomfort. I emphasised the potential negative effects of modern wheat and alcohol, and recommended avoiding wheat totally, using only ancient spelt wheat that is less reactive, also to limit alcohol intake.

A COMPREHENSIVE DIGESTIVE STOOL TEST WAS ORDERED

RESULTS:

Showed bacterial overgrowth. Pseudomonas aeruginosa was indicated, (a species of bacteria that often attacks the respiratory tract). There was no growth of healthy bacteria, Lactobacillus that reside in the small bowel and levels of beneficial Bifidobacterium species that reside in the large bowel, were low.

SUPPLEMENT PLAN RECOMMENDED FOR ONE MONTH:

- Probiotic Bifidobacterium powder, 2 doses daily with food
- Probiotic Lactobacillus species, 1 daily with food
- L-Glutamine powder, to heal the gut, 1 level teaspoon in water daily on empty stomach
- Slippery Elm Plus, to protect the gut, 1 daily 20mins before each meal
- Sea Plasma for nutrients and digestible protein, 1 daily with each meal
- Protein powder, as before
- Uva ursi tincture, antibacterial botanical, 15 drops three times daily, anytime of day
- Barberry Plus, antibacterial botanical, 1 dose twice daily on empty stomach
- Multi vitamin and mineral complex, 1 daily in middle of breakfast
- Brain Food formula, supplying specific amino acids for

enhanced brain function
* Soaked overnight flaxseeds for essential fatty acids to be taken at breakfast (anti-inflammatory and soothing on the gut lining)

MONTHLY FOLLOW-UP VISIT:

Responded well, drastic (Richard's words) improvement and he felt well again. Last five days feels totally fit with no gastric pain, brain 'fog' had cleared. I recommended completing one more month of supplementation to ensure he remained in good health, then to keep to good dietary balance to keep the gut healthy.

A TELEPHONE CALL, one week later, Richard had come down with shingles.

* Lysine-C was added to the treatment plan, 2 lysine (amino acid), a total of 1000mg/2gms vitamin C daily with food
* B Complex 50mg, 1 daily with breakfast
* Calcium/Magnesium/Zinc and malic acid formula, 1 level teaspoon daily in water anytime

The above programme to be taken for one month.

DIET:

To avoid nuts, chocolate, seeds, oats and carob (arginine-rich foods which compete with lysine) just while shingles was still active and whilst he was taking lysine treatment.

I advised if possible, to avoid long-term expensive protein supplementation, he might consider adding chicken and fish to his diet after he had completed the programme for shingles, as his lifestyle could benefit from this change, and I could not guarantee a future without any signs of ill health. Healthy immune function usually depends on adequate animal-based protein in some individuals and he had experienced a bout of shingles, a viral problem.

Richard mentioned he was willing to try, considering how well he felt with protein powder (dairy). He was adamant that wheat would stay out of his diet and he would be cautious with alcohol.

FINAL RESULTS:

He had recovered well from the shingles, had completed the supplement programme and felt very positive and healthy overall.

He was now eating chicken regularly, struggled a little with fish but would persevere for the sake of his health. He would also like to start cycling 60–80miles daily to train for charity rides.

He requested a sports nutrition multi formula, to support him during his proposed sport activities, preferred not to run a stool retest, and was then discharged feeling happy with the progress made.

CASE HISTORY FOUR

DARIO consulted me via Skype, email and with one personal visit. He was diagnosed with ulcerative colitis 3 years previously.

MEDICAL HISTORY:

- No other illnesses in previous years, apart from a history of frequent colds and infections, and recent infertility problems
- Family history of cancer and allergies

CLINICAL OBSERVATION:

Dario was on medication for ulcerative colitis, which over in the past three years had caused quite persistent bleeding with frequent loose stools, abdominal pain and intestinal inflammation.

Within the last four months, new medication was prescribed to slow down the faecal transit time; this was a successful treatment plan but the bleeding continued. He sweated profusely at times, and was constantly irritable.

He complained that stress makes the symptoms worse and certain foods also exacerbated the symptoms.

In the last 10 days he was prescribed cortisone, and the bleeding had subsided.

Joint pain and stiffness, arthritic type pains troubled him and he suffered with insomnia.

Dario had very low energy, and problems digesting fatty foods. He suffered with bloating and flatulence and experienced anal irritation. He ate under stressful conditions, and on the move, due to his occupation as electrician.

He suffered with backache in the lumber region, which had been constant for the past two years, but worse in the morning on waking. He had tooth decay, hair loss, dandruff, tingling hands, depression and nervousness.

He had an impatient nature, was achievement driven and he often got angry. Dario had difficulty getting to sleep and required over 8 hours sleep to feel ready for the day. He needed stimulants, tea and coffee to get himself going in the day, and often felt drowsy in the afternoon, and felt very sluggish all day.

Tests (due to finance) were not recommended. The damage in his gut was clear to see and needed urgent attention. Medication was managing to reduce severity of the symptoms but no healing was taking place.

CURRENT DIET:

- Tea, biscuits and yoghurt or tea, cake and fruit for breakfast
- Raw vegetables with white rice and fruit plus fish at lunch, or soup and white bread

- Had a need for frequent meals, was addicted to sugar, and was constantly hungry, dizzy and irritable when missing meals
- Took 4 coffees throughout the day with water in between meals, plus a cup of tea
- Normal table salt not sea-salt was added to food
- He drank alcohol, 2–3 glasses of wine per week, filtered water and did not buy organic produce
- Childhood diet was high in saturated fat and sugar
- Additives in food were not avoided, 3 teaspoons of sugar a day were added to coffee
- All food was washed prior to eating
- All grains products were processed white flour, he ate on average 15 slices of bread per week and a lot of pasta on most days, drank one pint of milk weekly and ate meat daily – both red and white

ASSESSMENT:

Suspected microbial infection, maldigestion, malabsorption. Increased gut permeability. Poor dietary balance, high sugar, processed food and stimulant intake, nutrient deficiency. Poor eating habits. Possible undiagnosed food intolerance.

The damage to the gut mucosal tissue appears severe, and will require a bland nutritious, healing, anti-inflammatory diet.

TREATMENT RECOMMENDATIONS

DIET:
- Avoid all dairy products, and gluten grains in any form
- Avoid tea, coffee, cocoa, alcohol, all sugar, biscuits, cake, wheat pasta, processed foods and food additives. Read labels carefully. Avoid red meat, pork, venison, smoked fish, barbecued meat, fermented foods, yeast, vinegar and strong spices
- Eat cooked vegetables, lightly steamed but not salad until matters improve. Avoid seafood, which due to their scavenging

habits could harbour bacteria

- Increase intake of dark green leafy vegetables, particularly green cabbage that contains vitamin U that heals ulceration, potato, garlic and onion soup that soothes and heals the gut
- An egg can be whipped into soup to add protein value. Plenty of root vegetables, cauliflower, onions, garlic for sulphur which helps heal the gut lining. Reduce fruits, eat only cooked sweet apples, fresh pears and sweet blueberries
- Use gentle anti-microbial herbs daily in cooking, thyme, oregano, basil and turmeric particularly to aid healing damaged tissue internally. Sage can help control sweating and rosemary and marjoram are astringent. Coriander, fennel and fenugreek can be very soothing. Take sea-salt but not table salt daily on food. This has a healing effect on the gut. Eat organic, where possible
- Eat plenty of protein for tissue renewal in the gut – light varieties that do not overburden digestive function, well cooked chicken, eggs and white fish, taking protein at each meal
- Avoid all cold meats that contain nitrites and sulphites, soya products, citrus fruits and very hot or cold foods that may irritate the gut
- Nuts could be eaten but not roasted or salted, they should be chewed well or ground. Large seeds can be eaten, provided they are chewed well, but not small seeds such as sesame that can become lodged in pockets – areas of the bowel that may become distended, damaged and inflamed
- Linseeds if soaked overnight and thoroughly ground have anti-inflammatory effects and helps healing of the gut
- If cravings for bread become extreme (as Dario mentioned may be the case) – home made flatbread, yeast-free, made with chestnut and chickpea flour or rice and buckwheat flour, sea-salt and olive oil can be enjoyed. Mashed potato whipped with eggs, and fried gently in avocado oil as fritters, can replace bread

- Unprocessed wholegrain rice, both as savoury dishes and rice pudding, made with rice milk, helps heal the gut. Rice milk can ease the gut pain. Advise never to re-heat food
- Not to become de-hydrated. Water should always be avoided at mealtimes but drunk throughout the day between meals. Avoid all fizzy drinks or fizzy water. Herbal teas that have soothing, healing effects are best, such as chamomile, liquorice, anis or cinnamon
- Improve breakfast balance with only cooked gluten-free grains, in rice, nut or coconut milk. This is easier on the digestion. Rice flakes with coconut and cooked banana, millet flakes with berries, ground almonds and coconut cream. Gluten-free oats can be eaten as porridge. Use fruit and cinnamon to sweeten
- Hard-boiled egg to follow at breakfast will help control blood sugar imbalance or a cooked breakfast with potatoes, eggs and mushrooms. Buckwheat pancakes with stewed apples and cinnamon are another option
- Avoid stress and take time to eat and digest

INITIAL SUPPLEMENT PROGRAMME FOR 3 MONTHS:

- Slippery Elm Plus, 1 taken 3 times daily 20mins before each meal
- Calcium, magnesium, zinc, 1 with each meal daily
- Male Multiple with amino acids, 1 taken at end of breakfast, to protect gut
- Multi formula nutrients to aid healing a leaky gut
- Omega 3 oil, Mega EPA oil, anti-inflammatory, 1 daily any meal
- High strength starflower GLA oil, anti-inflammatory, 1 daily any meal
- Mastik gum, heals ulcers and is anti-bacterial, 2 at bedtime on empty stomach
- Berberine and grapefruit seed, anti-microbial botanical, 1 mid-morning and 1 mid-afternoon on an empty stomach

FINAL RESULTS:

Dario felt well on this programme, improving slowly as time went on and noticing that symptoms were slowly clearing. The bleeding was less and the bleeding bouts were becoming less frequent, usually occurring only when he was stressed. He also recovered very quickly from these bouts, unlike in the past.

He tolerated all supplements very well, also all dietary recommendations, he was in fact enjoying his food much more. The only draw-back was, he was often offered his favourite dish – pasta, which he reluctantly had to refuse. I mentioned to him the option of buying gluten-free pasta made from lentils and rice.

Dario was keen to discontinue his medication and had voluntarily stopped the drugs for the first two weeks. He felt well. The third week he had stomach ache and diarrhoea, but no bleeding (which had always been the case in the past).

I recommended him to notify his doctor, explain his case and take advice, with a view to discontinuing his medication.

Dario explained he was advised not to stop medication at all, so he decided he would make his own decision on the matter, to add just one anti-inflammatory tablet on odd days when needed. This strategy worked well, until two brief flare-ups with diarrhoea and mild bleeding occurring two months down the line. The flare-ups were brief and cleared up rapidly. He felt well in the gut now, with no discomfort or pain and stools were normal and well-formed.

I recommended one month more on the supplements, then to rely on the diet, with instructions to be strict in the future on food and drink choices, as symptoms could return.

Reminding him he should look upon this as a permanent change in dietary habits, as his case was serious and had risks attached for his future health. He agreed he would do his very best as considering the progress he had made, he had experienced good effects from dietary changes.

CHAPTER FIVE

Digestive Disorders, Self-Help Treatment Plans

'The natural force within each of us,
is the greatest force in getting well.'
Hippocrates 460 BC

To achieve a healing process,
one needs to achieve the right mind-set.

Imagine you wish desperately to get well, you seek out the best practitioner, have total faith in their ability to treat you, but you were born with a rather laid-back attitude that prefers to leave important matters in the capable hands of others. You may not consider that you need to turn the best advice into an action plan where you are the main player.

YOUR HEALTH IS BASICALLY IN YOUR HANDS

Only you can turn your health around with the support of your practitioner. You are informed of the right conditions to initiate healing, the expert advice, how to formulate a plan for change but ultimately the rest is up to you. Slow progress occurs when a lack of participation creeps in.

You may have lack of time, be undermotivated to make all the changes required because despite feeling unwell, you enjoy your current unhealthy diet and the lifestyle, or you may feel the practitioner will take care of all the requirements needed to make you well again. Your mind-set may give rise to feeling natural health approaches mimic a drug prescribed treatment plan, where no or little lifestyle and dietary changes are recommended by your doctor and the medication miraculously heals you. Natural health care is an approach that is a partnership between patient and practitioner, it works with nature and is in tune with the body.

Follow instructions half-heartedly and you will get a half-hearted response. It has been proven in clinical practice time and time again, that with full compliance and cooperation from a patient, the desired outcome is achieved.

At this stage it should be obvious that by eliminating the factors that contributed to your poor health, it would be an error to return to those very poor habits again.

GENERAL DIETARY GUIDELINES FOR IMPROVING GUT HEALTH

The following changes to your eating habits will help you digest, absorb and utilise nutrients from your diet, improve your metabolism, revitalise your body, fight inflammation and start a process of healing. Only by taking away suspect foods and replacing with healthy options, can you move forward.

Once you feel in a consistent improved state of health, a more relaxed approach can be used, as some food items may be tolerated in irregular small amounts but always listen to your body; if it protests, there is a reason and you need to reduce or avoid this item, sometimes permanently from your diet.

AVOID:

All potential stimulating, inflammatory promoting and hormone disrupting foods: Black tea, coffee, cocoa or chocolate, caffeine containing fizzy drinks, undiluted pure fruit juice, alcohol, wheat, dairy and sugar.

SUGAR

Excess sugar in any form – honey, maple or agave syrup disrupts blood sugar levels. Once feeling well again, some people may tolerate limited honey or some other form of natural sweetener from dates, maple or agave but it is wise to avoid all cane sugar for life. It can cause so much disruption in body systems, is acid forming, has no nutritional value, contributes to vitamin and mineral deficiencies and is the cause of considerable health problems in the gut by providing fuel for pathogenic organisms. Zinc and vitamin B6 are essential for insulin production and blood sugar regulation, for hormonal balance and healthy skin and many other enzyme actions. Eating sugar can deplete your body reserves of these vital nutrients.

A glass of pure fruit juice delivers a large dose of glucose and fructose, fast releasing sugars into the bloodstream, that stress the pancreas and contribute to insulin dysfunction. It is far better to take your carbohydrates in a complex form.

Pulses, wholegrains, whole fruits and vegetables all contain various sugars that the body requires for energy but in contrast to extracted fruit juice, or a quick sugar fix, these foods contain valuable fibre and nutrients that slows down the entry of sugar into the bloodstream, it is then evenly metabolised without causing hormonal imbalance or sugar cravings.

Research, even back in the 1970's showed that as little as 6 teaspoons of sugar (the amount in a Mars bar or a large biscuit) reduced the effectiveness of immune white blood cells by 25% over a period of a few hours. This study also stated, that 24 teaspoons, the average amount of sugar in a banana split desert, can reduce, for many hours, white blood cell activity by a staggering 92%.[1]

White blood cells are your first line of defence against invading organisms so avoiding sugar can enhance immune function and help fight attack by harmful organisms.

ALCOHOL

According to nutrition lecture notes by Max, Schneider M.D. in 1995 from The University of California:

Alcohol inflames and irritates the lining of the gastrointestinal tract and impairs digestion by increasing stomach acid, reducing pancreatic enzymes, peristaltic movement and the absorption of nutrients in the small intestine.[2]

TEA, COFFEE, COCOA OR CHOCOLATE

Schneider also states that tea, coffee and cola drinks have been found to increase irritation of the stomach, cause irritability in the intestinal tract and malabsorption of nutrients.

The stimulating effects of coffee can result in depleted B vitamins, zinc and other nutrients from the effect on stress hormones. Considering how important B vitamins and zinc are in digestive function, once you are well again, it would be wise to limit coffee intake.

Both coffee, tea and cocoa contain stimulants, theobromine, caffeine and theophylline, which affect the central nervous system. Cocoa and tea stimulant levels, however are weaker than coffee. When suffering with digestive complaints, stimulants of any description, can cause discomfort, pain or irritation in the gut. Tannic acid in strong tea is particularly irritating on sensitive damaged tissue in the gut lining and it interferes with the alkaline minerals – calcium, magnesium and zinc absorption.

WHEAT

Modern varieties of wheat and other gluten grains have been shown to exacerbate symptoms of IBS. In an ION Study in 1994 on the effects of wheat on IBS, it was concluded that "Dietary manipulation is effective in IBS sufferers, and a high probability of prolonged symptomatic relief is achieved with elimination of suspect grain foods".[3]

Wheat in its modern hybrid form can be an irritant to the gut lining, it is also, due to the high gluten content difficult to digest and absorb, compared to traditional wheat varieties. It has been demonstrated to contribute to bloating, flatulence and discomfort in the gut.

AVOID:

All refined processed white wheat flour products and products made with sugar: biscuits, buns, cake, processed cereals, snack bars.

DAIRY

Dairy is a food designed to rear calves, not a natural food for humans who after weaning, are the only animal species who continue to consume milk, and this from another living species. Many studies show dairy intolerance to be implicated in IBS and other digestive conditions. A 2014 study concluded that "There appears to be consistent evidence that GI symptoms improve when milk is removed from the diet."[4]

Dairy is mostly pasteurised, homogenised and not a good source of calcium. Not everyone has difficulty digesting this food, but it is not to be recommended for individuals suffering with digestive complaints and indeed may be a contributory or leading factor in symptom development.

REPLACE WITH:

Unprocessed organically grown wheat-free wholegrains: sugar-free/wheat-free muesli, wholegrain wheat-free pasta, naturally leavened wheat-free bread, wild/wholegrain or Camargue rice. Use whole fresh fruits for sweetening baked foods, with sweet spices and coconut flower sugar. Eat healthy snacks if you need extra calories, oat or rice crackers with nut butter, fresh fruit, nuts, seeds, coconut flakes, sugar-free carob chocolate, nutritious dates and figs (not other dried fruit which is high in concentrated grape sugar but can instead be used for baking sugar-free cakes with cinnamon and coconut sugar).

Snacks are generally not a good idea when you have digestive problems – as the gut needs to rebalance and clear out between meals without a frequent input of food. However, if your activity load is high, then you may require the extra calories for energy output.

Natural sweeteners include – sweet spices, cinnamon, star anis, pure vanilla powder, cardamom, cloves, nutmeg, allspice and for more savoury dishes all green herbs, dill, caraway, saffron, turmeric, fennel seeds, coriander, sweet paprika, cumin. Many herbs and sweet spices have added benefit as they contain anti-inflammatory and anti-microbial properties.

Herbal teas have anti-inflammatory, anti-stress calming effects – chamomile, calendula, mullein, valerian, fennel, ginger, verbena or liquorice. (Avoid all mint teas, due to the tannin content.)

Mild chicory or dandelion root coffee may be tolerated where digestion is sluggish.

Carob powder, a nutritious cocoa substitute containing high levels of calcium, protein and fibre has a soothing effect or warm nut or rice milk diluted with water.

Warm organic apple juice diluted with ¾ water with/without cinnamon is very nourishing.

Low tannin open leaf herbal teas, red bush, Oolong, some mild Darjeeling, jasmine tea or mild green tea, should give you a comforting drink without irritating your gut. They all taste good with a little nut milk – particularly hazelnut milk, though this is a matter of preference. Teas all contain tannins in varying degrees; tannic acid binds alkaline minerals and make them unavailable to the body, so it is not the best idea to drink strong dark tea. Over time – deficiencies of alkaline minerals such as calcium, magnesium, potassium and sodium can develop. Try to make all teas mild, to enjoy the flavour without having a large dose of tannic acid, that lowers your mineral reserves. Avoid tea bags – they can have a detrimental effect on the gut, recent research points to the link with plasticide particles contained in teabags – even in non-bleached varieties. In my own organic shop years ago, a tea plantation owner explained the use of *'dregs'* – left over sub standard dust from leaves that is put to good financial profit in teabags. The quality nutrient containing leaves are sold as loose tea. I was sold! Especially as teabags with *dregs* are higher in tannic acid than loose tea.

AVOID:

Hydrogenated or partially hydrogenated (treated with hydrogen gas to stabilise) cooking oils or fats – these can be recognised as standard stabilised cooking oils on supermarket shelves, margarine or designer spreads with a mix of various fats and oils. These contain *trans fats* and can damage cells.

REPLACE WITH:

Avocado oil, olive oil, coconut butter used at low temperature. Use linseed, hemp oil or other cold-pressed unrefined oils to dribble on food but not to cook with. The best oil for gentle frying is avocado, it does not degrade at higher temperatures, though no oils should be highly heated. Trans fats can act as saturated fat and contribute to free radical damage in cells.

Some people may tolerate butter from cow's or goat's milk products, which contain valuable butyric acid – a main short chain fatty acid which provides a source of energy for new cell growth in the gut. This is essential for maintaining the integrity of the intestinal lining and helps probiotic colonisation. The nutritional value of butter is also high, with beneficial levels of vitamins A, D, E and K2, so where possible it is beneficial to continue eating butter. In good health humans produce short chain fatty acids from bacterial breakdown of dietary fibre.

AVOID:

Chemical additives in food: artificial colours, flavour enhancers, preservatives, emulsifiers, cosmetic waxes – there are literally thousands and thousands of chemicals in your food which should not be there. The food has been adulterated and can present a health risk. It is brought to the market in this state for a long shelf life, you could almost consider it 'dead' food, as it has little nutritional value. Also avoid the use of table salt which is not a healthy mineral condiment but contains sodium chloride.

REPLACE WITH:

Additive-free organic produce, natural organic herbs and sweet spices and condiments – pink rock salt, sea-salt or sea-salt with herbs. Herbal sea salt (Herbamare/Trocomare), is a healthy option containing well balanced levels of sodium and potassium – your electrolyte minerals vital for electrical activity in nerve cells. and some iodine for healthy thyroid function. It is not true that you should eat a salt free diet, it is table salt that is bad for your health, with high sodium levels. Mineral salts are a component of the human body. Your blood and tears contain salt. They are essential for contraction of muscles, supplying chloride to produce stomach acid, and to regulate the electrical activity of the body, especially the heart muscle. Without these electrolyte salts, being dramatic about it, the human body cannot survive.

AVOID:

Where possible non-organic produce. The pesticide and herbicide sprays that are used throughout the growing period on fruit and vegetables, can and do leave toxic residues on produce which end up in your body, despite washing procedures. These are dangerous persistent toxic chemicals that can disrupt your hormones and many of these chemicals have been found to be carcinogenic.

REPLACE WITH:

Organically grown seasonal fruit and vegetables, (out of season fruit and salad can be artificially ripened and is hard to digest) with natural organically reared meat, eggs, wild fish, and meadow reared dairy products, (avoiding produce using antibiotics and growth promoter drugs) that are still used in meat production and dairy farming industries despite world-wide exposure of the dangers to health through the food chain.

High fibre foods from pulses, nuts, seeds, grains, fruit, vegetables and salad promote healthy stool formation and elimination. Both soluble and insoluble fibre are contained in these foods – the elixir for the gut environment. Dark green leafy vegetables, rich in chlorophyll and magnesium, are extremely healthy for the body. Root vegetables are rich in minerals and healthy trace elements.

Once digestive health has been achieved, the occasional coffee, hot chocolate or alcoholic drink may or may not be tolerated, it is a question of individual constitution. These beverages are certainly harmful to the body at certain levels and have been proven to irritate the gut and upset digestive processes in individuals suffering with digestive disorders.

EAT YOUR WAY THROUGH THE RAINBOW

With fresh organic produce, colourful fruits, vegetables and salad – red, yellow, orange to blue, purple, black and all shades of green, vegetables can be lightly steamed, with a lid on to preserve colour and nutrients. Deep dark green broccoli, kale and chard are especially beneficial providing plant chemicals to protect cells – vitamin K, magnesium, vitamin A, calcium, folate, vitamin E, iron, B vitamins, vitamin C and manganese. The colour indicates nutrient content –

if produce is cooked to extinction, and pigments and flavonoids in the colour has been lost – powerful anti-oxidants with potent good effects on health have been destroyed.

If tolerated and when eaten before a main meal with a healthy oil dressing – a daily raw mixed colourful organic salad full of natural enzymes is beneficial in helping to stimulate gastric juices. Sometimes uncooked plant fibre is harder to digest when digestive function is compromised, so apply some caution with this advice. Salad may best be tolerated at midday instead of before an evening meal, this may also be the case with fresh fruits. One must pay attention to body signals and reactions until the digestive system is functioning well again.

TOP TIPS:

Cooking at a very high temperature destroys pigments, nutrients and denatures protein, making it harder to digest. Burnt or deeply browned barbecued fried foods can be carcinogenic and very unhealthy to consume. Steaming or cooking one pot dishes with a lid on helps to retain nutrients.

Re-heating food can create or contribute to bacterial contamination, causing more strain on digestive function. This is to be avoided until digestive function strengthens.

Always retain steamed water after cooking, this is rich in nutrients – so incorporate it into soups.

Avoid eating fruit directly after a protein rich meal; it could ferment whilst waiting for protein digestion to complete which is a longer process than for carbohydrate digestion. It is best to eat fruit at breakfast or alone between meals.

If eating out, make healthy choices from food that is freshly cooked with basic identifiable colourful ingredients, deserts without sugar, such as crepes with stewed fruit, baked banana with coconut and cream, or fresh fruit and crème fraiche. It may be possible to request your own choice of recipe.

Avoid drinking with meals as water which is alkaline will dilute your stomach acid. The stomach acidity needs to be very low, to stop infectious microbes from gaining entry to the gastrointestinal tract, and to help you digest your food efficiently.

Drink quality plain water, bottled or filtered tap water, regularly throughout the day and last thing at night. This helps overnight metabolic clearing processes, helping detoxification and elimination. It also sets the scene for passing regular, morning stools.

Water is required for all your metabolic processes. For blood fluidity, healthy circulation, and general tissue lubrication throughout the body. Every cell is bathed in fluid, if de-hydration sets in, brain function can deteriorate, thought processes can become muddled and body function can become sluggish.

Eat at regular times to keep your digestive hormones functioning well, they function best with a regular eating routine. Be relaxed and contented at mealtimes. Your gut will keep in good health with the right care and attention.

These dietary changes should provide relief from any distressing gastrointestinal symptoms.

I have occasionally been asked by some people, who, having achieved a successful treatment outcome with relief from all symptoms and improved digestion – as to when they can return to a 'normal diet'? The answer is – to prove a point, do a little trial – revert to old unhealthy habits and you will soon see that your symptoms invariably return, this is the most obvious, positive evidence of a cause and effect.

Unhealthy processed food is not 'normal' food in any sense, but sometimes old habits die hard, and the food industry giants continue to gleefully total up the profits from junk and designer foods.

SELF-HELP TREATMENT PLANS FOR DIGESTIVE DISORDERS
IBS – IRRITABLE BOWEL SYNDROME

This condition manifests itself in the entire gastrointestinal tract. It is a broad-based diagnosed gut disorder, covering a range of diverse digestive and bowel symptoms, but with no known pathology present and is a consequence of impaired digestion which occurs for variable reasons.

CAUSES:

- Dysbiosis (abnormal microbial balance in the gut), fungal/bacterial overgrowth. Parasite infection
- Lactose intolerance. Dairy intolerance
- Chronic stress, which can inhibit digestion
- Intolerance to wheat and/or gluten
- Low stomach acid (Hypochlorhydria) or lack of stomach acid (Achlorhydria) and pancreatic enzymes production
- Zinc and vitamin B6 deficiency, required for production of stomach acid
- Deficiencies of B vitamins, magnesium and manganese, required for digestive function
- Acid/alkaline imbalance
- A high sugar, processed food and alcohol intake
- Low water intake, becoming de-hydrated which increases tissue acidity
- Hurried mealtimes, eating under stressful conditions
- Chronic constipation and toxic bowel (retained old waste material, and lack of dietary fibre)
- Medication, especially NSAIDS, non-steroidal anti-inflammatory drugs, which can cause increased gut permeability, or antacids

EFFECTS:

Symptoms range from cramping, abdominal pain, alternating diarrhoea, constipation or loose stools, mucus in the stools, nausea, bloating, flatulence and loss of appetite, indigestion.

There may be food intolerance, allergies and sensitivities, indicating leaky gut.

IBS can develop into more serious disorders if left untreated. Compromised gut permeability can increase long-term risk of autoimmune disorders, including, rheumatoid arthritis, lupus, MS, and lead to fibromyalgia, chronic fatigue and inflammatory conditions.

DIETARY RECOMMENDATIONS:
Follow the general dietary guidelines on page 117.

Adapt to:

Avoid all grains apart from organic wholegrain rice, quinoa and gluten-free oats, (oats do not contain gluten but are often grown close to gluten grains, causing cross contamination. Soya milk, red meat and seafood or sushi with raw fish.

Additional foods to add in to help soothe and heal the gut:

Cabbage, especially savoy and dark varieties. Potatoes, baked, lightly roasted with avocado oil or boiled but not fried. Rice pudding made with sugar-free rice milk or nut milk and cinnamon. Wholegrain rice flakes. (Contains gamma oryzanol which helps gut healing.) Coconut products. Ground linseeds and hempseed on breakfast cereal, providing anti-inflammatory essential fatty acids and protein.

Eat light protein sources, chicken, eggs and fish, sulphur containing foods, cauliflower, onions and garlic which are beneficial in healing the gut lining. Make soups with these foods plus potato and cabbage and beaten eggs, taking care not to re-heat food. Chew all food well.

RECOMMENDED FUNCTIONAL MEDICINE (FM) TESTS:

(Always with the advice of a Functional Medicine practitioner or Clinical Nutritionist.)

- Gut Permeability
- Comprehensive Digestive Stool Analysis with parasitology
- Food Intolerance
- Specialised Wheat Gluten Reactivity & Autoimmunity panels

RECOMMENDED SUPPLEMENTS:

- Multi vitamin mineral formula with high dose B vitamins
- Zinc as gluconate or citrate and vitamin B6
- Psyllium husk product, high in fibre and mucilage – helps cleanse the bowels
- Gentle plant based digestive enzymes with low dose HCL (hydrochloric acid)
- Berberine and grapefruit seed botanical product (anti-microbial)
- L-Glutamine powder – the primary nutrient source for the small intestine, helping to heal the gut
- Multi-strain non-dairy probiotic
- GLA essential fatty acid (anti-inflammatory)

GENERAL ADVICE FOR SUPPLEMENTATION:

Always start initially with low dose remedies which enables the body to utilise nutrients and botanicals at a rate best suited individually for efficient metabolism; work with the body not against it, watching for significant signs, both positive and negative. Usually your body will indicate how it feels. There will be a lot of biochemical changes occurring whilst on treatment plans, it is not always the case that progress goes only forward, it is quite normal for improvement to fluctuate as the body systems work hard to achieve nutritional balance or eliminate undesirable bugs. Work with the signals it gives out and adjust accordingly. There is no overnight magic cure; it takes a long time to develop chronic digestive disorders and it can take in some cases a long time to reverse them. Often matters are straightforward and progress is made rapidly with positive benefits seen within weeks.

Seek medical advice if on medication, some herbal formulas are contra-indicated with certain drugs.

The above programme is appropriate for a period of 1–3 months. Providing you are doing well, a decision can be made to continue the programme, minus the anti-microbial product, it is not appropriate to take botanical anti-microbial treatment long-term, without professional assessment.

If there are still health problems, you should seek practitioner advice. If the measures recommended in this book as self-help do not entirely clear up your health issues, then there may be other underlying unidentified causes that need to be addressed.

LIFESTYLE RECOMMENDATIONS:

Get plenty of sleep, rest and put effort into establishing a regular sleep routine to keep hormonal balance. This will help achieve deep-seated healing from restorative sleep. Participate in non-competitive enjoyable outdoor exercise. Walking, cycling or swimming is ideal, though the latter, whilst health is poor should be avoided as there are many negative effects from chlorinated water. Some pools do however use other healthier options to disinfect the water such as the ozone or ioniser methods of water purification. Avoid vigorous activity and all stressful situations where possible. Meditate or practice yoga. Read, enjoy warm baths with essential oils and reduce your computer time.

FOOD INTOLERANCE AND ALLERGIES

An allergy is an immune reaction to a food or environmental allergen. The immune reaction occurs when the body perceives the invading substance as an invading organism and a chain of reactions occur, including histamine release as the body overreacts to the situation and this can produce a wide range of symptoms.

A permanent atopic allergy will always involve the immune system, a cell mediated response which produces an Ig E antibody reaction. An Ig E antibody reaction usually presents with an immediate onset of symptoms, these antibodies in the blood can be measured after a challenge from the antigen (the offending food or substance).

CAUSES:

- Lectin, a protein known as glycoprotein, found in many foods can activate an immune response in susceptible individuals, and is sometimes implicated in allergy and auto-immune disease
- Sulphites and nitrate food additives can also provoke an immune response. Toxic residues which can remain on produce following intensive farming spraying practices
- Polluted pollens and mould in the atmosphere
- Gut dysbiosis and poor detoxification

A permanent allergy can be a life-threatening situation. and may cause anaphylactic shock that comes on immediately after eating the offending food. Most likely suspect foods are peanuts, fish, shellfish, eggs, soya milk and wheat.

EFFECTS:

Symptoms vary, between shortness of breath, wheeziness, constriction of airway passages and lowered blood pressure, to hives and skin rashes.

When the microbiome (the bacterial balance) in the intestinal tract represents an unhealthy environment, digestive processes are affected and can lead to food intolerance and increased gut permeability, increasing overall the likelihood of immune reaction.

It is not always the food at fault but the state of health of the host body. Once healthy, a person can sometimes re-introduce problem foods, even with true allergies, particularly if the incidence of original allergic reaction occurred as a one off due to food contamination, but this approach needs expert advice, to help differentiate between permanent allergy to natural chemicals present in foods and the environment and inability to handle microbial or toxin contamination due to a person's poor detoxification processes.

Food intolerance, in contrast is a sensitivity to natural or toxic substances which does not normally involve the immune system in its response, it is non-atopic food reaction and symptoms usually come on gradually rather than instantly, becoming evident as a delayed reaction. Sometimes this reaction can occur up to three days or so after exposure to suspect foods, making it extremely difficult to identify where the problem exists in the overall eating pattern.

It involves a non-immune response. Food sensitivity can occur when any of the factors mentioned under 'causes' of IBS, are evident. When the gut is healthy, sensitivity usually does not occur. It is the body's response that tells you all is not well and apart from identifying and eliminating problem foods, action should be taken at the same time to assess the state of the gut and measures taken to improve the gut environment.

EFFECTS:

Symptoms can range from bloating and flatulence, stomach cramps, distension, nausea, vomiting, stomach pain, loose frequent stools, headache, persistent cough, itchy skin and heartburn.

Chronic nutritional deficiencies may develop and contribute to other signs of poor health; fatigue, a tendency to frequent infections, forgetfulness, depression, irritability, anxiety and hormonal disturbances.

These are signals that indicate 'problems ahead'! and need prompt action because if left unattended these symptoms may develop into more serious disorders.

DIETARY RECOMMENDATIONS:
Follow the general dietary guidelines on page 117.

For advice when not choosing to test for food intolerance:

All meals should be noted in a food diary and all suspect food reactions carefully noted. Cover at least a period of one week to include potential delayed reaction time to food.

If suspect foods are noted, a dietary plan should be formulated to eliminate all items that may present a problem, choosing healthy alternatives from the dietary guidelines. An elimination-challenge diet should then be put in place for between 3–6 months, and all measures taken meanwhile to eat a healthy diet, improve your digestive function and heal your gut.

After the elimination period, the challenge part of the diet is necessary to see – if having improved your digestive health – you can now tolerate these certain foods again.

Re-introduce the suspect foods singly for a period of 1 week for each item tested. Eat more than a normal amount of the food item.

Note any negative reaction and any increase in pulse rate. If there is no adverse response, include the food item back into the diet. If a negative response is experienced, continue to avoid the offending food for a further 1–3 months. A digestive enzyme product may help to introduce a food back into the diet but if after time there is no improvement in the sensitivity experienced, testing procedures may be at this stage a consideration or the option made to remove the food permanently from the diet, provided it is not a main category of food as this will require careful replacement of healthy alternatives to maintain a balanced dietary intake.

Sometimes eating a main food category in a different form can improve matters, a good example is the case of modern hybrid wheat intolerance. Modern variety of wheat is very indigestible and has a high gluten content, traditional non-hybrid strains of wheat with a lower gluten content, such as spelt are nutritionally superior to modern wheat and can be much better tolerated, providing digestion is functioning well.

If cow's milk dairy gives you problems, a trial with goat's milk products which have a lower protein content, are easily digested and are better tolerated, can often bring good results.

Should you prefer to opt for a test for food intolerance, it is necessary to be eating the suspect food for at least between 6–8 weeks. This action is required to evoke the immune response, that is being measured. Antibody production can only occur if the antigen (suspect food) is present in the body. As previously mentioned, test procedures should be undertaken with professional guidance.

RECOMMENDED FM TESTS:

- Comprehensive Digestive Stool Analysis and Parasitology
- Food intolerance
- Gut permeability

RECOMMENDED NUTRITIONAL SUPPLEMENTS:

- Multi vitamin mineral with high dose B vitamins, to aid digestion
- Zinc and vitamin B6, for stomach acid production
- Vitamin C with bioflavonoids, with anti-histamine and anti-inflammatory effects
- Magnesium citrate, to reduce stress, relax muscles and aid digestion
- Essential fatty acids GLA, EPA to reduce inflammation
- Calcium citrate, to calm the antibody-antigen binding reaction
- Plant based enzymes and HCL with pepsin, to help digestion

- L-Glutamine powder, to aid repair of intestinal lining
- Probiotics to reduce colonisation of pathogenic organisms

If bloating or flatulence exists

Add botanical herbs, artemisia, berberine, garlic, oregano, echinacea, grapefruit seed oil for a month, until the problem clears.

LIFESTYLE RECOMMENDATIONS:

If this is an issue, reduce stress in your life, eat under restful calm conditions for all meals. Chew all food to a pulp and do not drink with meals. Get as much sleep as you can, rubbing lavender oil on the abdomen before bed and take regular gentle exercise that can benefit the gut in many ways. Do not overtax the body mentally or physically as this can interfere with optimal digestion.

GASTRIC AND DUODENAL ULCERS

Ulcers may be gastric, duodenal or occasionally oesophageal. They are caused by a break or lesion in the epithelial lining of the gastrointestinal tract, which becomes ulcerated and destroys localised tissue. Acid contents from the stomach irritate and inflame the area, gastric emptying is delayed and in the case of gastric ulcers, bile may back up from the small intestine to the stomach.

CAUSES:

- Chronic gastritis, inflammation of the stomach lining
- Overconsumption of tea, coffee and alcohol. Smoking
- Prolonged stress and anxiety
- Medications
- Nutritional deficiencies and poor dietary balance

EFFECTS:

- Griping intense burning pain on an empty stomach, which is often relieved by eating
- May include, heartburn, distension, nausea, vomiting, weight loss, diarrhoea, perhaps blood in stools if it is a bleeding ulcer
- Poor appetite and excessive salivation

DIETARY RECOMMENDATIONS:
Follow the general dietary guidelines on page 117.

Adapt to:

- Avoid all gluten grains, chicory or dandelion coffee
- Raw potato and cabbage juice (savoy cabbage) contains potassium and vitamin U which has healing properties for all types of ulcers. Eat cooked potatoes in any form (not fried), to soothe the gastric lining. Dark green leafy vegetables, root vegetables, avocados, celery, cucumber, courgettes, pumpkin, squash, carrots, cauliflower, sprouts, cabbage, chard, and beetroot (without vinegar) can all be enjoyed when gently steamed
- A bland alkaline based diet, that does not irritate the damaged area is advised. No strong spices, no acidic fruits or salad items such as tomatoes. Bananas, pears and melon and ripe grapes and blueberries are ideal
- Coconut products can be eaten and rice or almond and other nut milks
- Unprocessed whole-grain rice is beneficial, and gluten-free oats or rice flakes cooked as porridge for breakfast, with a little unblended pure honey for healing inflamed tissue. Ground almonds, hemp and linseed, for healthy fats can be sprinkled on top but not cooked
- Eat light organic protein, plenty of eggs, for choline to help gut

repair, white fish (not smoked or seafood) and well-cooked chicken. Protein and healthy fat is needed to heal ulceration and to renew tissues

• Eat varied green herbs and garlic in your food to help treat infection and use sea-salt for healing purposes, this is good for wounds and for relieving inflammation, by balancing acidic conditions in the tissues

FM TESTS

None recommended, if a medical diagnosis has been made.

RECOMMENDED SUPPLEMENTATION:

• Mastic gum, to help eradicate bacteria. This is effective against Heligobacter Pylori, a bacterial infection that has found to be linked to intestinal ulceration

• Slippery elm, marshmallow and gamma oryzanol from rice taken before meals, to relieve pain and protect the gut lining from food

• Pure aloe vera capsules, to aid healing

• L-Glutamine powder, an amino acid (protein) required for cellular growth in the gut lining

• N.A.G. N-Acetyl Glucosamine, a potent amino sugar to aid healing. This is a component of mucous membranes throughout the body, it forms the gel-like structure between collagen fibres

• Phospholipids from lecithin to assist in relieving stress in nerve tissue and to maintain structure of cell membranes

• Vitamin A and zinc for tissue renewal in the mucous membranes of the gut

To replace taking a multi vitamin and mineral supplement that could irritate the area, organic spirulina powder, sprinkled on savoury food will supply a range of all nutrients plus high levels of protein, in a gentle easily absorbable form to aid tissue healing and support metabolism.

LIFESTYLE:

- Try to avoid stress, eat in a calm manner, meditate and be early in bed to rest and allow healing to take place
- All meals should be well chewed to help digestion as it is not appropriate to give digestive support in the form of enzymes or hydrochloric acid

GASTRITIS

This condition describes inflammation of the stomach lining without ulceration.

CAUSES:

- Medication
- Infections
- High or low stomach acid
- Poor digestion
- Acute stress that can set off an attack. Chronic stress that can contribute to development of the condition

EFFECTS:

- Intermittent throbbing pain which sometimes migrates up into the oesophagus. Often worse during the night, there may be appetite loss and a nervous stomach, constipation or diarrhoea and weight loss
- Possible vitamin B12 deficiency, the cause of pernicious anaemia
- Possible iron deficiency, which can cause anaemia

RECOMMENDED FM TESTS:

- Food intolerance
- Gut permeability
- Comprehensive Digestive Stool Analysis with Parasitology
- Adrenal stress

DIETARY RECOMMENDATIONS:
Follow the general dietary guidelines on page 117.

Adapt to:

- Avoid all gluten grains, and any form of tea, even herbal. Tea, alcohol or coffee or any refined food, can irritate the gastric lining in sensitive individuals
- Drink sugar-free rice milk to relieve the pain. Bananas which are rich in potassium are also beneficial in alleviating the throbbing pain
- Stay on the bland alkaline diet mentioned on page 136 with plenty of eggs for choline and protein. As pain subsides and you feel more comfortable, you can relax the diet to include other healthy items
- Gastritis tends to fluctuate in intensity and frequency and often follows a period of stress or eating habits that set up a resistance inflammatory response. If you become aware of this, it is possible to foresee circumstances and take avoiding action
- With time, patience and nurturing of the gut, gastritis can subside and become a problem only when the gut is challenged through extreme chronic stress or poor dietary habits

RECOMMENDED SUPPLEMENTS:

- Follow the above nutritional supplement advice for ulceration but exclude mastic gum and add GLA/EPA/DHA essential fatty acid to help reduce inflammation
- If infection is present, a choice of cinnamon, garlic, oregano, thyme or cloves, in a food-based oil form, a couple of drops diluted in water daily, have an antiseptic effect

LIFESTYLE:

Stress plays a large part in controlling bouts of gastritis, achieving a relaxed attitude will allow the digestive system to heal, improve and function well again.

Once you have experienced gastritis, it is wise to avoid excessive strong tea and regular alcohol intake especially wine and spirits. Avoiding sugar and very strong spices such as chili will help to ensure your gut heals for good.

HIATUS HERNIA

A condition that describes protrusion of the stomach, above the diaphragm, and can affect the junction between the gullet and the stomach. A hernia is a protrusion through a weakness in the abdominal wall, it can be shown externally as a lump in the groin or on the abdominal surface.

In hiatus hernia, the oesophageal valve is affected by pressure, and remains open allowing food and acid to be regurgitated, causing GERD (gastroesophageal reflux).

CAUSES:

- Weakness of the diaphragm muscle, from injury, or pressure from heavy lifting

- Obesity
- A low intake of fibre in the diet
- Overeating
- Mineral deficiency or imbalance, required for muscle tone (calcium and magnesium)

EFFECTS:

Heartburn, burning pain behind the sternum, made worse by bending or lying down.

DIETARY RECOMMENDATIONS:

Follow the general dietary guidelines on page 117.

Adapt to:

- Follow a bland alkaline diet mentioned on page 136. Keep food portions small, chew well and eat slowly. Hydrate well between but not with meals, food material should be moist and well-formed, not compacted
- Raw potato juice can help the discomfort. Rice milk can help to relieve the pain. Porridge made with rice flakes and milk and a little quality honey can give some comfort, especially at suppertime. Make the last meal of the day small and easy to digest. It is preferable to eat the main protein meal of the day at lunchtime
- Avoid all meat, eat eggs and fish until symptoms subside. When improvement is felt add in light meat to the diet
- Eat plenty of root vegetables for fibre but avoid grains apart from cooked millet, oats and rice

RECOMMENDED SUPPLEMENTS:

- Slippery elm, marshmallow and gamma oryzanol, soothes and reduces inflammation by protecting the digestive wall with mucilaginous compounds. These can also help promote growth of beneficial gut bacteria
- Psyllium fibre formula with gentle plant digestive enzymes can help to break down the food, the fibre helps the passage of food through the gut and provide soft bulking material to help relieve pressure on the intestinal tract
- Powdered organic spirulina and chlorella, for nutritional support
- Powdered chelated magnesium and calcium to help improve muscle tone

LIFESTYLE:

Sleep propped up with pillows. Avoid all lifting and heavy carrying. Take gentle exercise to improve muscle contraction. Massage abdomen with essential oils that help relaxation. Lavender oil warm baths can reduce tenseness and aid sleep.

COLITIS AND ULCERATIVE COLITIS

Colitis is inflammation of the lining of the colon, the large bowel.

Ulcerative colitis describes a condition when ulcers have formed in the colon.

CAUSES:

- Microbial infection
- Poor dietary choices
- Poor digestion and toxic bowel syndrome
- Lack of fibre and an inflammatory promoting diet

- Food intolerance and stress

EFFECTS:

In Colitis:
- Frequent diarrhoea, pain and cramps in the lower abdominal area
- Discomfort, bloating, and flatulence on passing stools

In Ulcerative Colitis:
- Frequent diarrhoea with blood and mucus and abdominal pain and discomfort
- Fatigue and lack of energy
- Symptoms may be mild, or severe in both conditions

RECOMMENDED FM TESTS:

- Comprehensive Digestive Stool Analysis with Parasitology
- GI Effects Microbial Ecology profile
- Food intolerance
- Allergy
- Adrenal stress
- Gut permeability

DIETARY RECOMMENDATIONS:
Follow general dietary guidelines on page 117.

Adapt to:

- Eat a bland diet, and take small portions as mentioned above, ensuring complete mastication so that undigested food material is unlikely to lodge in the intestinal lining. Avoid all grains except cooked rice, gluten-free oats and millet. Avoid small seeds such as sesame or chia that can likewise become lodged in the gut lining. Pumpkin and sunflower seeds ground or well chewed would be best. Linseeds should be taken only when completely ground

- Eat a fibre rich diet – plenty of steamed root vegetables and potatoes in every variety, dark greens, well chewed salad items and fruits, avoiding pineapple, uncooked apples and citrus fruits. Blueberries, bananas and pears, mangoes and grapes would be best but not to be eaten after a protein meal. These fruits combine well with nuts and seeds for essential fats and cooked grain and eaten at breakfast. Cooked stewed apples with cinnamon powder can relieve diarrhoea or eaten with rice pudding made with rice milk, it can be soothing and nourishing and would be tolerated well as a dessert, taken 1 hour after waiting for a protein-rich meal to digest

- Avoid red meat and pork or venison, if poorly digested, this can linger in the bowels, putrefying and causing infection. Heavier meats take longer to digest than light alternatives such as lamb, chicken or turkey. Avoid fried foods, these can irritate the gut

- For ulcerative colitis, a high protein and fat diet is indicated to enable tissue healing, so eating fish (not seafood or smoked fish) and plenty of eggs is beneficial, plus lighter protein. These provide building blocks for ongoing tissue renewal in conditions with ulceration

- Eat plenty of healing herbs and garlic on all food to help disinfect the gut, together with sea-salt, but avoid all strong spices and fermented, vinegar containing products

- Baked potatoes can be very soothing for the potassium content and if tolerated with melted butter

- Keep the diet well-balanced. Keep well hydrated between meals

RECOMMENDED SUPPLEMENTS:

- Mastic gum, antibacterial aid
- Slippery elm, marshmallow and gamma oryzanol taken before meals soothes the gut
- Berberine and grapefruit seed formula, anti-microbial aid
- Multi vitamin and mineral formula capsules only, provides general nutrition
- Bifidobacterium non-dairy probiotic, support for the large bowel
- DGL liquorice, the glycyrrhizin which promotes potassium loss is removed in this product. It is anti-inflammatory and has healing properties on the gut mucosa
- L-Glutamine powder, As the main fuel for the gut cells, to aid healing
- N.A.G. N-Acetyl Glucosamine to support connective tissue healing
- Aloe vera without benzoic acid added, this supports the healing process
- Vitamin A and zinc which play a role in strengthening connective tissue and for cell tissue renewal
- As the healing process progresses, gentle plant enzymes (in the middle of meals only) can be added to improve digestive function

LIFESTYLE:

- Avoid stress, have plenty of relaxation and early bedtimes to help healing processes
- Ensure restful mealtimes, paying attention to dietary choices that are easy to digest. Gentle exercise that does not tax the abdominal muscles

CANDIDA AND FUNGAL OVERGROWTH

This condition is caused by an overgrowth of yeast. It may be localised or systemic, which is referred to as it's mycelial form, when it can quickly invade many parts of the body.

There are many species of fungi; Candida albicans is one of the most common species, found in the human gut, it resides there normally without a problem but can become overactive under certain conditions and cause fungal health problems.

CAUSES:

- High intake of sugar and refined carbohydrates
- Overuse of antibiotics
- Medications
- High alcohol intake, which feeds fungi
- Toxic heavy metals, such as copper, which promotes fungal overgrowth
- Copper can become elevated in the human body with synthetic hormone use from the pill and HRT
- Copper sulphate used as a fungicide and sprayed on fruit and vegetables, can also enter the human body

EFFECTS:

- Bloating, fatigue, backache, flatulence, brain fog, irritability, bowel disorders, sugar cravings, rashes, itchy skin, thrush, PMS, cystitis and frequent infections
- There may be evidence of fungal toe nails, or fungal patches on skin or in the mouth
- Food intolerance, joint pain, muscle aches, poor memory, blurred vision

RECOMMENDED FM TESTS:

- Yeast culture

- Comprehensive Digestive Stool Analysis with Parasitology

DIETARY RECOMMENDATIONS:
Follow the general dietary guidelines on page 117.

Adapt to:

- Maintain strict avoidance of sugar in any form (honey, fructose, sucrose, glucose, syrup, dextrose, lactose, and molasses and dried fruit (a concentrated sugar). Some low sugar fruits such as tart apples and berries, (sorbic acid in berries has anti-fungal effect) are acceptable, to avoid experiencing low energy levels. Avoid all fruit juice. Use sweet spices for sweetening, sugar-free jams and apple juice and lemon juice
- Avoid all yeasted products – bread, marmite and added yeast in ready-made products
- Avoid all fermented products; vinegar, pickles, alcohol, soya sauce, mayonnaise. Use herbs, garlic and ginger to flavour foods. Olive oil has anti-fungal properties and should be used daily. Cured, smoked foods should not be eaten
- Avoid spicy foods, blue cheese, mushrooms
- Enjoy yeast-free, wheat-free bread varieties
- Oat cakes and rice cakes are fine, also buckwheat pancakes, millet, wholegrain wheat-free pasta and sugar-free, wheat-free muesli
- Enjoy goat's milk products, yoghurt and cottage cheese, plenty of fresh salads, vegetables, organic eggs, meat, fish, beans and pulses, seeds, coconut, (contains caprylic acid with anti-fungal properties)

RECOMMENDED SUPPLEMENTATION:

- High dose garlic, which has anti-fungal properties

- Biotin which inhibits the conversion of yeast to the mycelial form
- Grapefruit seed extract which has anti-fungal properties
- Multi strain probiotic, to improve microbial balance
- Caprylic acid, echinacea, Pau d'Arco, olive leaf, black walnut and oregano are a few of the many herbs that exert anti-fungal effects
- A high dose multi vitamin mineral product (free of yeast)
- Vitamin C which has antimicrobial effects

LIFESTYLE:

- Plenty of rest, exercise and fresh air. Do dry skin brushing to help the lymphatic system remove waste such as dead yeast from cells. Our skin is the most important largest organ of elimination
- Take warm essential oil baths, which help to disinfect and promote circulation. Drink plenty of water to help detoxification

COELIAC DISEASE

Severe intolerance to gluten in wheat, rye, barley grains, causing changes in the mucosal lining of the small intestine. This disorder occurs at any age.

CAUSES:

- Undiagnosed food intolerance
- Impaired digestion
- Can be triggered by stress, surgery, or infections

EFFECTS:

- Severe malabsorption of nutrients in untreated coeliac disease, due to a damaged gut lining from flattened villi, small finger-like projections that support absorption in the small intestine

- Widespread nutritional deficiencies, causing potential multiple symptoms of ill health
- Upset bowels, IBS, lassitude

DIETARY RECOMMENDATIONS:
Follow the general dietary guidelines on page 117.

Adapt to:

- Be totally gluten and dairy-free (butter or goat's products should also not be included). Dairy intolerance can be experienced with gluten sensitivity. Attention should be given to food variety, colour and balance, replace dairy with options given in information on dietary advice
- Non-gluten grains such as gluten-free oats, buckwheat, rice, corn, millet should be used, but preferably cooked. Sweet cinnamon, anis or cloves can help to flavour food with a small amount of coconut sugar. Baked apple, pears or banana complement grains at breakfast. Ground nuts and seeds can be sprinkled over when serving
- Protein and healthy fat is required to provide building material to repair the gut
- The diet should be rich in easily digested light protein, eggs, poultry and white fish and healthy fat from nuts, seeds and oily fish such as salmon or trout. Avocado, coconut and olive oil can be used in cooking
- Linseed oil provides vital EPA, DHA and GLA essential fatty acids when converted by enzyme action in the body, although this action is inhibited by stress, ageing, tobacco and alcohol use or high intake of processed oils containing omega 6 fatty acid. Linseeds or flaxseeds contain valuable levels of fibre that benefit the gut, the oil can be used cold to dribble on food
- Light pulses, lentils, peas, mung beans and small black beans provide fibre to help peristalsis, the movement of food along the digestive tract, and many vitamins, minerals and some amino

acids for cellular repair. Soaking pulses overnight and discarding the water, then rinsing well helps the body to digest these foods

- All food eaten should be light on the digestive system, small meals, colourful and nutritionally well balanced. Omelettes with mushrooms or herbs provide a perfect protein that is easily digested. Vegetable soups sprinkled with spirulina and hemp powder, helps to increase the protein content and further provides vitamins, minerals, trace elements and essential fatty acids

- Cooking practices should favour steaming with a lid on pots to help maintain nutritional value. Wholegrain and wild rice meals and starchy root vegetables with legumes and lentils supply healthy carbohydrates for energy production as the body needs to work harder to digest and absorb food when the gut lining is damaged

- Citrus fruits may irritate, so eat with caution. Ideally bananas, berries, pears, grapes, mangoes and stewed fruits would be best. Salads contain natural plant enzymes which help digestion, but they will need to be chewed well and used with healthy oil dressings to help absorption

RECOMMENDED FM TESTS:

- Gut permeability
- Food intolerance
- Comprehensive Digestive Stool Analysis and Parasitology
- Coeliac and gluten sensitivity panel
- Wheat/Gluten Reactivity and Autoimmunity Screen
- Vitamin B12 and iron status should be evaluated by a professionally trained practitioner

RECOMMENDED SUPLEMENTATION:

- Slippery elm, gamma oryzanol and marshmallow to soothe the gut before eating

- L-Glutamine, to provide fuel for healing the gut
- N.A.G. N-Acetyl Glucosamine for gut repair
- Vitamin A, to strengthen intestinal tissue, support immune function and to maintain health of the gut lining
- EFAs, essential fatty acids to aid healing. GLA, DHA and EPA omega oils have an anti-inflammatory effect
- Zinc and vitamin B6, to improve digestion
- A food state multi vitamin and mineral capsule formula plus spirulina powder to replenish nutrients, particularly B vitamins needed for healthy skin. The spirulina provides readily absorbed pre-digested protein, a valuable source of amino acids to be used as building blocks for improving villi structure
- Broad spectrum digestive plant enzyme formula, to help malabsorption. Caution should be given; start as a trial in the case of severe discomfort. The enzymes should be tried in the middle of each meal, just one daily to start. When tolerated they will ease digestive strain and help the body's task of metabolising your food efficiently
- Vitamin C which is required with zinc for new skin growth should be taken only in a buffered form as magnesium or calcium ascorbate and not on an empty stomach
- A quality multi strain non-dairy probiotic to aid absorption and help re-build gut flora

LIFESTYLE:

Reduce stress and allow time for good digestion. Be strict in food choice and you will benefit from improved gut health.

CROHN'S DISEASE

This condition affects mainly the lower part of the small intestine. It involves a thickening of the gut wall, which produces obstruction and ulceration in the intestinal mucosa.

CAUSES:

- Poor digestive function
- Viral and bacterial infections in the gut
- A high refined carbohydrate and sugar diet

EFFECTS:

- Swollen abdomen, severe abdominal pain, vomiting, diarrhoea, weight loss, fever, lower GI bleeding, cessation of bowel movements and bowel fissures
- Malnutrition due to poor absorption
- Can cause stunted growth and delayed puberty in children

DIETARY RECOMMENDATIONS:

Follow the general dietary guidelines on page 117.

Adapt to:

- Ensure that protein from light protein sources is increased in the diet
- Avoid all sugar forms and refined grain carbohydrates, all gluten grains, all dairy, red meat, pork and venison
- Avoid tannins in tea and in herbal teas, keep well hydrated
- Do not re-heat food
- Eat an alkaline based diet, rich in fruits, root vegetables, pulses and lots of green leafy vegetables to provide fibre, nutrients and increase peristalsis. Cook all non-gluten grains, use rice or nut milk and rice, nuts and ground seeds. Eat eggs, chicken and fish, particularly oily fish salmon and trout. Protein and fat is required for renewing damaged tissue but should be in a form that the body can digest easily
- All strong-tasting food or drink items such as hot spices, vinegar, flavourings, un-ripened fruit, tart apples, citrus

fruit should be avoided. The delicate gut lining can be very sensitive and needs some nurturing with gentle flavours that do not represent a challenge on painful tissue

- If an issue, to maintain weight calorie intake should be increased. Small, regular, balanced (carbohydrate/protein/fat) meals or snacks should be taken every 2 hours, taking care not to overtax the body
- Use herbs, onions and garlic liberally in cooking to reduce risk of infection and provide sulphur for detoxification and healing
- The diet should be well-balanced to ensure adequate nutrition

RECOMMENDED FM TESTS:

- Comprehensive Digestive Stool Analysis with Parasitology
- Comprehensive Parasitology as an alternative to help identify infection
- Food intolerance
- Gut permeability
- Vitamin B12 and iron status should also be professionally evaluated

RECOMMENDED SUPPLEMENTATION:

- Dairy-free broad-based probiotic capsule
- Mastic gum, anti-bacterial agent or berberine, or artemisia botanicals
- Anti-microbial oregano oil as a recommended dose on the container, taken internally
- Slippery elm with marshmallow and psyllium husks, to soothe the intestinal tract
- Gamma oryzanol from rice to relieve discomfort
- A high dose multi vitamin and mineral formula in a powdered form

- Vitamin C in buffered form to aid fissure healing as calcium, magnesium ascorbate. If constipation or difficulty passing stools exists, an increased level of vitamin C is required, but only in the magnesium form
- Zinc sulphate or gluconate in liquid or powdered form for support in mucosal lining healing processes
- Magnesium citrate increases peristalsis by muscle relaxation and helps the passage of food material through the gut. This works well with vitamin C to help loosen stools
- Liquid vitamin A to aid healing the gut lining
- Low dose plant enzymes, taken in the middle of meals, to help digestion
- EFAs (GLA and EPA) for anti-inflammatory support
- L-Glutamine powder, a powerful healing agent for the gut
- N.A.G. N-Acetyl Glucosamine to support gut healing

DIVERTICULITIS

This disease is characterised by the formation of pockets or pouches in the large bowel. The pockets can become infected by pathogenic microbes or become inflamed due to trapped faecal material.

CAUSES:

- Disturbed peristalsis
- Constipation and dehydration
- Lack of fibre in the diet
- Poor muscular toning in the large bowel
- Incomplete digestion

EFFECTS:

Symptoms can include; nausea, vomiting, abdominal distension, colic, general malaise, chills, fever, cramps, diarrhoea, and difficulty eliminating stools. Incomplete healing can produce fibrosis and narrowing of the colon.

RECOMMENDED FM TESTS:

- Food intolerance
- Gut permeability
- Comprehensive Digestive Stool Analysis with Parasitology

RECOMMENDED DIET:
Follow the general dietary guidelines on page 117.

Adapt to:

- Eat gluten-free grains, rice, corn, millet, buckwheat, and gluten-free oats
- Cook all grains, gradually increase fibre rich foods to help bulk the stools
- It is vital to avoid constipation
- Carob powder drinks rich in dietary fibre can be beneficial
- Increase fruit and vegetables and eat ground nuts only, not seeds as these can become lodged in intestinal pockets causing inflammation. Increase green leafy vegetables for magnesium, which helps relax muscles, eat root vegetables and pre-soaked well-cooked pulses. Fruits would be best taken stewed until symptoms improve
- Avoid salads until symptoms improve
- Hydrate well, throughout the day. Drink organic carrot juice to provide vitamin A for healing
- Use plenty of herbs, garlic and onions in dishes
- All food should be chewed to a pulp. Eat meals in peace and quiet

RECOMMENDED SUPPLEMENTATION:

- A multi nutrient formula with spirulina, chlorella plus greens in powdered form, for general nutrition
- GLA omega 6 and EPA/DHA omega 3 oils, as anti-inflammatory agents
- L-Glutamine powder, for healing the gut
- N.A.G. N-Acetyl Glucosamine for healing the gut
- Vitamin C powder as an antibacterial agent, together with zinc powder to heal the gut
- Liquid vitamin A for support of the epithelial lining in the gut
- Magnesium citrate to soften stool formation and aid peristalsis
- Echinacea tincture, as anti-microbial agent
- Oregano oil (at recommended dose)
- High dose multi species probiotic to re-colonise and balance gut bacteria

There are many different herbal therapy options; the recommendations mentioned above represent the botanicals I have used successfully, over the years.

Researchers in one article commented that the use of herbal therapy in inflammatory bowel disease is increasing world-wide.[5]

This article published from the University of Athens Medical School, highlights the benefit shown in clinical trials, from herbal therapy for Crohn's disease and ulcerative colitis, using mastic gum, artemisia, boswellia, aloe vera, curcumin, wormwood and tormentil.

The role of L-Glutamine is well established in supporting health of the epithelial lining in the gut.

The epithelium serves as a barrier to entry from toxins, allergens and pathogens. In a leaky gut, the lining is open to these noxious substances, which can cause inflammation and tissue damage.

In one study in the US, researchers concluded that... "In small bowel mucosa, Glutamine is a unique nutrient, providing fuel for metabolism, and repair and maintenance of the gut barrier function".[6]

RECOMMENDATIONS FOR MINOR DIGESTIVE COMPLAINTS AND RELATED SYMPTOMS

BLOATING AND FLATULENCE

This complaint arises from incomplete digestion when undigested matter can be fermented by bacterial action and produce various gases which move around the intestinal tract. It is commonly related to a high intake of sugar and processed white flour products, which provide food for unhealthy species of bacteria allowing them to multiply at a fast rate. Processed foods also lack adequate levels of nutrients, required for production of stomach acid and digestive enzymes. In time this can give rise to poor digestion, and gut dysbiosis (imbalanced gut flora). Odorous unpleasant flatulence indicates incomplete breakdown of food by digestive enzymes and unabsorbed material passing into the large bowel.

If you digest well and your food choices are healthy, you should have a relatively flat stomach, feel comfortable after meals, and experience no bloating or flatulence. If you are unable to reach a happy outcome with advice in this book, it would be best to seek the advice of a professionally trained nutritional practitioner.

SELF-HELP:

Reduce overall your carbohydrate intake. These sugar-containing energy foods ferment easily, particularly starches in the form of pasta, beans, bananas, potatoes and white rice. Avoid alcohol, fizzy drinks, chocolate, biscuits, cake, all bread, sugar in any form and high sugar-containing fruits, such as grapes, pineapple.

For snacks replace with:

• Wholegrain rice or oat crackers with hard cheese and apple, or nut butter
• Citrus fruit, nuts, seeds and figs

- Eating protein and fat with carbohydrates can help stop sugar cravings

Increase protein in each meal and reduce the carbohydrates. Root vegetables and potato starches can provide an energy source if eaten with an adequate helping of protein and should be eaten in the correct portions, to maintain satiety and a feeling of comfort. Avoid complete carbohydrate meals taken without protein, such as a bowl of chips with salad and pizza without any protein, fish, cheese or meat as this equates to feeding the body high levels of sugar. Eat colourful organic fresh food with plenty of green vegetables.

SUPPLEMENTATION:

- Take HCL and pepsin, 1 capsule with main meal and any other high protein meal
- Plant based digestive enzyme formula 1 before each meal
- A quality high dose B vitamin multi vitamin mineral formula 1 with breakfast
- Chew all food to a pulp and do not drink with meals. Eat under peaceful conditions taking ample time to digest your meals

CONSTIPATION

This complaint arises from a poorly balanced diet with inadequate fibre and fluid content such as that provided by fresh fruit, salads and vegetables, together with nuts, seeds, whole grains and pulses. Constipation can also occur with a high intake of animal protein, which unless balanced with the correct ratio of unprocessed fresh plant foods, takes longer to digest and is a heavier type of diet which slows the transit time; the rate the food passes through the gut.

A diet with a higher carbohydrate content with lighter foods, rich in fruit, vegetables and greens, that digest easily is required together with a choice of lighter protein and regular water intake, particularly last thing at night to help elimination in the morning. Taking a little apple juice in a glass of warm water can hydrate at a slower rate than pure water, ensuring less night-time disturbances for the bladder.

Peristalsis depends on good levels of calcium and magnesium for contraction and relaxation of muscles.

Exercise and movement daily helps this action, sitting for long periods hinders it.

Constipation can also occur with a diet that is low in magnesium-rich foods (nuts, wholegrains, dark green leafy vegetables), and inadequate vitamin C intake (fresh fruits, vegetables and salad).

SELF-HELP:

- Increase intake of soluble and insoluble fibre, making sure you eat a wide variety of these fibre rich foods, a variety of fruits, green leafy and root vegetables, colourful salad, wholegrains, beans, peas, lentils, nuts and seeds. All greens contain chlorophyll which is a magnesium containing pigment, and highly nutritious
- Hydrate throughout the day with quality plain water with a dash of lemon. Walk briskly at least one hour per day or take regular exercise twice daily. This can help the peristaltic movement in the intestinal tract that moves faecal material along the gut with wave-like motion in preparation for elimination
- Take a daily warm bath or shower with rosemary bath milk and rub essential oils such as rosemary which increases circulation, on the abdominal area. Magnesium oil can also be applied in the same way before bed. Lavender bath milk and oil can be beneficial in helping muscles to relax

SUPPLEMENTATION:

- Take 1–3 grams of vitamin C (ascorbic acid) twice daily with water. This dose can be varied to suit individual metabolism; the upper level should be adequate to reach bowel tolerance levels. These levels are contra-indicated with women using the Contraceptive Pill or for individuals on anti-coagulant medication. If in doubt, refer to your doctor

Vitamin C is water soluble, and non-toxic, it will help to loosen the stools and improve elimination and improve peristalsis. When this has been achieved the dose can be reduced to 1-2 gram daily to keep the bowels healthy and cleanse the intestinal tract. Vitamin C has many values, it is anti-inflammatory, anti-microbial, anti-oxidant (protecting cells from damage by oxidation in normal body processes) and is necessary for efficient immune function and absorption of some minerals

- 400–600mg of magnesium citrate daily. When stools become regulated this dose can then be reduced to 200mg daily in the evening. Magnesium relaxes the muscles throughout the body and helps to induce a feeling of calm. It de-stresses the body and is required for digestive processes
- Two tablespoons of golden linseeds (not ground) pre-soaked overnight, with your breakfast. Add 1 tablespoon of psyllium husks (wheat-free), be sure to drink water 1 hour after breakfast and regularly throughout the day, to help flush the material along, but not with the meal as it can interfere with digestion
- Slippery elm and marshmallow products to help provide mucus forming material to protect the gut lining, whilst supporting the regulation of bowel movements

LOOSE STOOLS, DIARRHOEA

This complaint can commonly occur with microbial infections in the gut. They can gain entry when stomach acid is low and the microbial flora in the gut is imbalanced. Lack of beneficial healthy bacteria to fight infection, promotes this situation. Yeast, bacterial or parasitic infections cause the body to attempt to eliminate the organisms and in doing so, the transit time of food is increased. The stools then become loose or diarrhoea occurs. Malabsorption can be a possibility as the food material does not linger long enough in the small intestinal area where absorption of nutrients takes place.

Treatment options for identified microbial infection have been mentioned earlier in this chapter, but meanwhile helping to slow the transit time and firm up the stools is beneficial. Anti-microbial treatment and tests for diagnosis should only be undertaken with practitioner advice.

Loose stools can also occur with a diet that is low in calcium content (wholegrains, dairy, vegetables, nuts and seeds). Phytate and phosphorus in foods can reduce absorption and a high intake of alcohol, or tea can interfere with reserves in the body.

SELF-HELP:

- Increase fibre rich foods, the material in the intestinal tract needs firming up, this will help to cleanse and eliminate toxins or unhealthy bacteria. Apple – particularly stewed apple can help to slow down the transit time, pectin is released and is beneficial together with soluble and insoluble fibre, for helping to bulk up the stools
- Avoid all hot spices, such as chili or curry. These spices are anti-microbial but could provoke an immediate response as your body attempts to eliminate, and in doing so, increases transit time again as unhealthy bugs are destroyed. Avoid acidic, fermented foods, vinegar and yeast
- Avoid all gluten grains, fizzy drinks, stimulants; alcohol and tea and coffee and eat a diet rich in pulses, root vegetables, green vegetables and wholegrains, protein at each meal and healthy fats
- Avoid dairy, focus on other calcium rich foods that have a high calcium to phosphorus ratio, kelp, carob, kale, parsley tea, all green vegetables, sesame seeds, endive, green barley

powder, figs, plus calcium rich sardines, pilchards, whitebait, salmon, chickpeas, almonds, black and pinto beans, sesame seeds, prawns, spinach, baked beans

- Temporarily reduce fruit except cooked apples, pears and bananas. Cook all wholegrains. Porridge oats and millet are best cooked with nut milk and sprinkled with nuts and seeds
- Eat plenty of herbs and garlic with antiseptic properties. Onion soup is very beneficial for infections

SUPPLEMENTATION:

- Take 500mg of calcium carbonate daily, split in two doses 250mg each, mid-morning and towards the evening but not with meals. This form of calcium is not well absorbed, but it does do the job of firming up the stools and slowing the transit time. When ideal stool changes are noted it would be best to switch to a calcium citrate, chelated or gluconate form if you plan to continue with calcium supplementation for health reason, bearing in mind that magnesium supplementation is also required as a co-factor for absorption as well as vitamin D and K.

PAINFUL ABDOMINAL CRAMPS AFTER EATING

Inflammation in the gut can be due to many conditions including bacterial or other microbial infections, food intolerance, indigestion, hormonal imbalance or arising from a high intake of acid forming foods such as drinking coca cola, carbonated designer drinks, alcohol or strong tea with high tannic acid content.

Pain, acid conditions in the body and heat all go hand in hand. Recommendations in this book provide information on diagnosed digestive disorders and how to find professional help. All symptoms relating to pain or cramps should be medically investigated before applying the following advice.

SELF-HELP:

- Avoid all dairy, sugar, alcohol, fizzy drinks, tea, coffee and gluten products
- Eat a bland diet rich in light protein such as organic chicken and eggs, plus salmon and white fish
- Avoid smoked fish and cold meats
- Cook gluten-free oats with rice milk for breakfast, add ground almonds and coconut
- Avoid dried fruit, keep to ripe pears and cooked apples until situation improves
- Eat root vegetables and well steamed greens with potatoes or wholegrain and wild rice
- Steam or bake food, do not fry
- Take one tablespoon of flaxseed oil with breakfast (not heated)
- Eat walnuts and almonds, sunflower and pumpkin seeds

SUPPLEMENTATION:

- Take one plant based digestive enzyme in the middle of each meal
- One low dose multi vitamin mineral capsule with breakfast
- Marshmallow and slippery elm powder before meals

HEARTBURN, REFLUX, INDIGESTION AFTER EATING

This condition can arise with hurried mealtimes, inability to relax whilst eating, incomplete mastication of food and being stressed whilst trying to digest food. Obviously focus should be directed, if this is the case, on dealing with these issues.

Heartburn or a feeling of fullness and discomfort after meals can also occur when stomach acid levels are low and insufficient pancreatic digestive enzymes are produced. There can be many reasons for this deficiency, most of which are discussed in former chapters.

Correct dietary balance is important, so as not to put added stress on digestive function; eating a large portion of meat and animal fat without the necessary vegetable fibre or starch can be hard to digest, equally, large portions of carbohydrate starches without some protein and fat can upset digestion. Carbohydrate, protein and fat balance in each meal should contain a correct balance of nutrients which helps the body break down your food more efficiently. Eating protein with each meal can help you store glucose more efficiently and balance blood sugar levels.

Think of the consistency and composition of your food, is it hard to break down, are you taking in drinks or food choices that your gut may rebel against? Such as alcohol, water or juice with meals.

It is also a good idea to listen to your body`s response to certain meals, you should feel comfortable in the gut with a feeling of satiety after a suitably balanced meal.

SELF-HELP:

- Avoid drinking at mealtimes (alcohol included). Take time for eating and for meals to digest well. Avoid coffee post meals, instead opt for calming herbal teas, chamomile or fennel
- Avoid eating piping hot foods or icy cold foods
- Eat small frequent meals, avoid over eating. Chew well

SUPPLEMENTATION:

- Take HCL and pepsin before each protein meal and 1 digestive plant enzyme formula with each meal
- A high dose multi vitamin and mineral product at breakfast

PERSISTANT MUSCLE ACHES AND PAINS

A condition that can be associated with dysbiosis in the gut and bacterial or parasitic infection. This would need investigating with a professionally trained practitioner.

Microbes create by-product toxic material that can be reabsorbed and systemically distributed throughout the body. Leaky gut syndrome and poor detoxification may also be a possibility. Practitioners can offer FM tests to check for infection.

SELF-HELP:

- Take herbal remedies for potential gut infections. Always check with your doctor for compatibility with any prescribed medicine you may be taking. If symptoms do not improve, I recommend practitioner advice
- Berberine, artemisia, grapefruit seed, oregano or thyme oil offer anti-microbial benefits
- Include cloves, cinnamon and garlic in cooking, as well as a variety of green herbs. Eat oily fish several times weekly

SUPPLEMENTATION:

- Take a multi strain probiotic to be taken at a separate time from the herbs
- A quality high dose multi vitamin mineral product
- 400mg of magnesium citrate daily with meals split in a morning and evening dose
- An essential fatty acid formula containing EPA/DHA/GLA with any meal containing fat to help absorption and reduce inflammation
- Vitamin C 1–3 grams taken daily in split doses. This has an anti-inflammatory effect

BLOOD SUGAR IMBALANCE – SUGAR CRAVINGS

Healing the gut and clearing up digestive disorders requires attention when dealing with sugar cravings. Sugar intake feeds bugs and disrupts blood sugar balance, it needs to be avoided at all cost.

Cravings usually occur when nutrient deficiencies exist, particularly chromium which is a key component together with vitamin B3 of glucose tolerance factor, which is released when blood sugar rises. Chromium and other B vitamins are found in wholegrains, vegetables, eggs, nuts and together with zinc, support healthy blood sugar levels.

Poor dietary balance with a high intake of processed white flour products and regular consumption of stimulants such as tea, coffee and alcohol or tobacco, can predispose a person to the development of fluctuating blood sugar levels. Being continuously dehydrated can also contribute to blood sugar imbalance. Regular tea drinkers also risk fluid loss through the diuretic action of tea.

When wholegrains known as complex carbohydrates, are eaten, they take hours to be fully digested, due to the wholegrains containing a lot of fibre, these are slow-releasing carbohydrates and should be favoured at all times. The glucose in the germ structure is slowly released and reaches the bloodstream in a consistent regulated action with excess glucose being stored in the liver and muscles for reserve energy needs.

In contrast, when simple sugars in the form of processed white flour goods, lacking nutrients or fibre and any sugared products enter the bloodstream, this is metabolised in a rapid fashion which causes a quick rise in blood sugar levels, leading to an energy increase, which some people find desirable in this modern hectic world. However, there is a risk of a subsequent dip in blood sugar levels a few hours later with cravings setting in, and the wish to repeat the whole process for the quick energy 'fix'.

Having balanced blood sugar levels from a healthy diet, relieves stress and supports function of all body systems.

SELF-HELP:

- Drink water regularly throughout the day. The body requires water to store glucose
- Avoid all stimulants and sugar
- Eat wholegrains for breakfast with protein in the form of sugar-free muesli, nuts, seeds and yoghurt or eggs and avoid all processed cereals. All pasta and rice should be in an unprocessed wholegrain form which retains all nutrients
- Cinnamon has been shown to improve glucose utilisation, this could be sprinkled on grains
- Add protein and healthy fat in some form at each meal, this slows down the rate of carbohydrate absorption
- Eat a diet rich in vegetable varieties, with plenty of dark green leafy items
- Find alternatives for a snack such as wholegrain crackers with cheese or nut butter, fresh fruit with nuts and seeds. Do not skip meals, eat regularly and take a snack when required between meals

SUPPLEMENTS:

- Take a high dose multi nutrient product at breakfast, specifically designed for blood sugar control, or a vitamin mineral product that has high levels of B vitamins in the range of 50mg of each nutrient as well as effective zinc levels of 20–30mg, chromium at 200mcgs, vitamin C at 500mg, magnesium at 200mg and manganese 2.5mg, plus the full range of other nutrients. These recommendations represent only approximate guidelines.

Supplementation choices vary with practitioners, if you experience severe uncontrollable sugar cravings, then you require professional assessment.

STRESS, ANXIETY AND TENSION

Stress will always impact negatively on digestive function as digestion switches off under stressful situations.

Walking daily, having regular sunlight and exercise and indulging in music and reading can help calm the mind.

An absorbing hobby or massage sessions with essential oils can all aid relaxation.

Nutrient deficiencies can contribute to anxiety and stress, particularly pantothenic acid vitamin B5, required by the adrenal glands in the stress cycle, and other B vitamins, zinc, vitamin C, magnesium, calcium. Vitamin B6 and zinc deficiencies have been linked to panic attacks and feelings of anxiety.

Stress causes the adrenal glands to produce hormones such as adrenalin which signals the liver to release glucose stores for energy action and prepares the body for fight or flight, as was required from the onset of civilisation. Digestion switches off, the hormone cortisone raises blood sugar levels, blood pressure and heart rate increases. Other hormones are released which help retention of sodium required for nerve and muscle activity. Chronic stress impacts health from all angles. Repeated increased metabolic rate which takes place during stress can lead to multiple nutrient deficiencies. As stress depletes the calming alkaline minerals calcium, magnesium and zinc and leads to excretion of other vitamins and minerals, particularly potassium, body systems dependent on these nutrients can develop serious disorders. One such system at risk is the nervous system which requires magnesium, sodium and potassium for efficient nerve transmission.

Hormones contain protein and fat. Any stressed individual does not require high levels of carbohydrates in their diet but increased levels of protein and fat, which have a calming effect on metabolism, digestion and nerve activity.

SELF-HELP:

- Drink water regularly, dehydration can cause mental and physical tension
- Ensure a daily exposure to sunlight or light. Do not use sunblock cream as this can reduce conversion of vitamin D from sunlight. Alternatively limit time in hot sun
- Eat a high protein and fat diet. Amino acids, building blocks from protein are required for neurotransmitter production to support health of the nervous system and are required for the structure of all cells. Essential fatty acids from healthy fats, polyunsaturated, monounsaturated and saturated, are part of the structural building blocks in the brain and in every cell membrane throughout the body
- Avoid all simple carbohydrates as sugar and focus on slow releasing energy foods
- Avoid all stimulants; tea, coffee, chocolate, alcohol, tobacco
- Eat a nutrient rich diet which contains a full range of nutrients specifically supplying support for the nervous system; nuts, seeds, wholegrains, vegetables, greens, fish, seafood, oily fish, meat, eggs, chickpeas, lentils, dairy products, potatoes, bananas, oranges, mangoes, berries, avocado, mushrooms, pumpkin
- Increase the following choline rich foods for brain food and to help control stress:

Egg yolk, nuts and seeds, especially sunflower, pumpkin, and almonds, salmon, seafood, poultry, broccoli, peanut butter, chickpeas and organ meats.

SUPPLEMENTS:

- Take a multi vitamin mineral product containing high dose B vitamins
- 30mg zinc citrate or gluconate

- Vitamin C 1–3 grams daily spread over the day
- 500mg of chelated calcium and magnesium 1:1
- Phosphatidyl choline and phosphatidyl serine from lecithin to support healthy fat metabolism, nerve and cognitive function

(Checking vitamin D levels may be indicated if exposure to sunlight is limited.)

FATIGUE AND LOW ENERGY

Foremost the diet should contain the nutrients the body requires to keep healthy and sustain energy. The body does not get sick due to lack of a drug, it gets sick through lack of nutrients.

The body runs on nutrients contained in the calories in your diet.

Secondly the food needs to be digested well and the nutrients efficiently absorbed.

Nutrient deficiencies can contribute to lack of energy. Energy production in the cells depends on a range of nutrients including vitamin C, magnesium, copper, CoQ10 and B vitamins.

If the diet is poorly balanced and the fuel for the body, the nutrients, are absent or in short supply, then the body will struggle to produce energy at the level necessary for a full day's activity. What would be the benefit of eating starchy pasta with tomato sauce as calories to fill the stomach, if it wasn't nutritionally balanced with vegetables, cheese, fish or meat?

Lack of restful sleep can also affect energy levels and it is hard to make up for lost sleep as the body has an inbuilt clock regulated by hormones. This circadian rhythm of life regulates energy and health. A lack of sunlight daily reduces vitamin D conversion on the skin. Vitamin D, known as the 'sunshine' vitamin is required for immune support and increasing calcium absorption in the gut. It is recognised for maintaining a stable nervous system.

An accumulation of dietary or environmental toxins can slow down energy production as the body struggles to eliminate harmful substances.

Microbial infection and gut dysbiosis can also affect cellular energy production. Areas best investigated by a professional.

SELF-HELP:

- Eat a nutrient rich varied diet, with a focus on fresh enzyme rich fruits, vegetables and salads
- Reduce fat and protein in the diet and eat energising carbohydrate foods, wholegrains that are rich in B vitamins with colourful fruit, vegetables and salad
- Avoid all stimulants, drink organic vegetable juices daily
- Get regular restful sleep, exercise but not excessively and ensure plenty of natural sunlight for vitamin D

STRESS, AND THE VAGUS NERVE

The vagal nerve is one of the largest nerve systems in the body. It stretches from the brain and wanders all over the body through most organs down to the lower abdomen. The main function of the nerve is to convey messages from the brain to the gut, and the gut to the brain, in a feedback loop system.

It is part of the parasympathetic branch of the Autonomic Nervous System and relaxes the body by keeping homeostatic function under control, by returning the body to peace and calm after 'the storm' of an adrenalin rush from the sympathetic branch of the nervous system. The body always attempts to maintain balance and equilibrium.

What significance does this have for you? Well…as the body returns to its 'rest and digest' (parasympathetic) mode following a period of adrenalin rush and stress, the vagal nerve is always involved in this action. It controls anxiety, your level of stomach acid production, and your stress levels and is linked to every aspect of digestive processes.

It appears to do this by friendly gut bacteria directly stimulating nervous system neurons to send signals to the brain. The gut microbes can produce hormones and neurotransmitters and the vagal nerve is the transport mechanism to 'talk' to the brain, via these hormones and neurotransmitters. In one study, researchers produced evidence that human gut organisms can activate the vagal nerve and help to promote good digestive health.[7] An indication that the microbiome is the central player in gastrointestinal health.

VAGUS NERVE ACTION IN DIGESTIVE HEALTH

The vagal nerve helps to manage all the complex processes going on in your gut, it signals muscles to contract and push food down the intestinal tract, releases acetylcholine a calming neurotransmitter that reduces inflammation, and helps to improve digestive function.

In another acclaimed Swiss study in 2014, investigating gut instincts, researchers concluded that the stomach has a say in how we respond to stress and anxiety and that optimal vagal nerve tone regulates stress and maintains digestive health.[8]

STRESS, DIGESTION AND THE HPA AXIS

The body controls mental, physical and emotional stress through a feedback system in the HPA axis, a major part of the neuroendocrine system involving the hypothalamus, the pituitary and the adrenal glands. They control the stress cycle by a series of chemical signalling reactions, which take place in response to stress, producing hormones to instruct the glands to increase or to decrease hormonal output.

The HPA axis system regulates digestion, immune function and your body's reaction to stress. When stress occurs, the body requires glucose to produce the energy required to fight the stress. In dealing with this normal reaction digestive processes are switched off when adrenalin and blood sugar levels rise as the body prepares for action.

Cortisol is the stress hormone released by the adrenal glands. When cortisol levels are high, receptors in the hypothalamus and pituitary gland release further hormones in a feedback system, signalling the adrenal glands to automatically lower cortisol, calm the body down and return it to a pre-stress state, a normal homeostatic function. The body always strives to maintain equilibrium and balance with very delicate hormonal and nervous system series of control.

The stress reaction in the body is completely normal, however when abnormal and constant levels of stress hormones are being produced in a frequent state of 'red alert', the adrenal glands themselves can become exhausted, causing dysfunction and what is recognised as adrenal fatigue – a disorder linked to chronic stress.

With chronic ongoing un-resolved stress, your digestive function will certainly suffer, and any degree of gut healing effort made, could be hindered until the stress issue is dealt with successfully. Chronic stress affects the total physical and biochemical ability of the body to maintain good health, so full progress in your programme can only be achieved by addressing and restoring balance in all body systems.

CONTROLLING STRESS

This obviously is an important aspect of healing and a considerable factor in your ability to reverse your health problems. Foremost, one should identify any abnormal stress response and try to reduce or remove the cause of your distress. Stress relieving food, drinks and therapies mentioned later can be used to aid control.

CAUSES TO CONSIDER:

LACK OF SLEEP is the most major cause of stress in the gastrointestinal tract.

The human body regenerates itself at night during sleep. Deny the body a few hours of this precious time, over regular periods and the sleep hormones will become disturbed, causing poor digestive health, insomnia and an increased susceptibility to infection.

You may have noticed at some time, when you were deprived of sleep, you were prone to picking up colds and infections.

Our circadian rhythms are a fundamental feature of all living things on earth. Our inbuilt body clock is regulated by our hormonal system. Hormones manage our wake-sleep pattern and our gut clock which regulates the level of digestive hormones, the secretion of stomach acid, the nutrient absorption in the small intestine, our immune function and antibody production, as well as gut motility and the maintenance and protection of the mucosal barrier.

According to a scientific review, published in The Journal of Physiology and Pharmacology in 2011, researchers concluded that disruption of circadian physiology due to sleep disturbance could account for various gastrointestinal disorders, including IBS, gastrointestinal reflux disorder, peptic ulcer, and increased gut permeability. They also found in studies involving melatonin (the sleep hormone), that it offered a protective mechanism on the gut mucosa, reduced inflammation, had positive effects on the de-sensitisation of irritated tissue, and relieved abdominal pain and distension.[9]

As there is constant connection between our gut and brain, sleep restriction or deprivation can cause chronic disruption in our gut feeding rhythms, and our ability to digest and absorb food efficiently. So, there is every good reason to ensure you have a good sleeping pattern of regular, same time in bed routine, as this is the only way your body clock can recognise when to produce the sleep hormones required for deep restorative sleep.

There is a knock-on effect in the gut if melatonin levels drop and mealtimes are not routinely planned as this can disrupt digestive hormones and contribute to gut disorders.

Deficiencies of the sleep hormone melatonin and excess levels of the stress hormone cortisol produced by the adrenal glands in the stress response, have been shown to play a large part in increased gut permeability or leaky gut syndrome. A recent research article, also states that poor sleep patterns and deprivation of sleep can negatively affect the microbiome in the gut.[10]

Another study concluded, with the fact that "sleep abnormalities contribute to gastrointestinal diseases, and conversely gastrointestinal diseases can lead to sleep disturbances." The researchers also found that Crohn's disease patients had 75% more incidence of active disease when also suffering with sleep disturbances.[11]

STIMULANTS IN THE DIET

If the gut is healthy, and you have conquered and dealt with your digestive disorder, a daily coffee or tea may be fine. However, it is not generally accepted by some members of the public that these beverages interfere with sleep patterns. They contain stimulants that cause a nervous system adrenalin response. Usually heavy tea and coffee drinkers experience sleep problems. The fact that you feel your body doesn't react in this way is testament to the body's ability to adapt. A stimulant is a stimulant and ultimately your body may enjoy more relaxing alternatives rather than being put in a state of *alert stress* throughout the day.

IMBALANCED BLOOD SUGAR LEVELS
CAN CONTRIBUTE TO STRESS

Eating foods containing complex carbohydrates, can mean more stamina, sustained long-term energy and improved glycogen storage (glucose reserves from diet are stored in the muscles and liver). This is not the case with refined simple carbohydrates that *flood* the body with sugar (refined white flour grains).

The sugar load from complex carbohydrates is gradually released over a few hours, due to the high fibre content. Foods to regularly include in your diet, are wholegrains (not modern wheat), pasta, rice, millet, oats, pulses and legumes.

Eating a carbohydrate snack later in the evening can help induce a healthy sleep pattern, sometimes sleep is disturbed simply because your blood sugar levels have dropped in the night due to a high intake of refined carbohydrates. A banana (which improves serotonin levels) or a little wholegrain oat porridge can help aid sleep.

Drinking sufficient water can also help to balance blood sugar levels. Never skip meals, make sure, if you are prone to blood sugar drops during the day, you have regular snacks every couple of hours, as this causes less stress on the body.

Intensive exercise before bed is not ideal either, as this activity can also disturb sleep patterns. If you are involved in endurance training of any description, the stress on the body can be extreme. By having the best supportive diet and some sports nutritional supplementation, the toll and stress on body systems can be reduced. Gentle exercise before bed and regular daily exercise outdoors, reduces stress and can help digestive processes.

KEEPING ACID ALKALINE BALANCE

Stress, what acidic foods we eat and how hydrated we are can shift our healthy slightly alkaline body into an acidic stressful state. This shift triggers the body to draw alkaline minerals, such as calcium from the bones, plus magnesium, sodium and potassium from tissues and organs, which act as 'buffers' to help reduce the acid and relieve the stress. This mineral loss in buffering processes for chronic acid tendencies can cause mineral deficiencies.

Pathogens can also proliferate in acidic conditions in the gut. Bacteria, viruses, yeasts or parasites produce acid waste products, that add to the load. Nearly all degenerative diseases have been linked to acidic conditions in the body.

Other conditions linked to acidic conditions in body tissues include, digestive problems, inflammation, poor immune response, bone loss, anxiety, stress and infections.

With alkaline conditions, there is improved digestion and immune function, good bone density, less infections, a calmer mental outlook and usually no inflammatory processes.

A healthy person's pH level should be between 7.1 and 7.4. You can test whether your diet is well-balanced in favour of alkaline foods by testing with saliva or urinary strips bought in the chemist. (Do not put saliva strip in mouth but spit on a saucer.) Test for five days before bedtime. (Do not brush teeth prior to test.)

Maintaining alkalinity is vital for good digestion and efficient function of body systems.

Alkaline foods come from the plant kingdom and acid foods from the animal kingdom. The acid or alkaline ash of metabolised foods is due to the content of various elements in the food. Either calcium, magnesium, potassium, sodium as alkaline elements in foods or phosphorus, sulphur, chloride as elements from acid forming foods.

All foods contain a mix of elements but it is the level of dominating elements that determine the acid or alkaline ash that is left after the metabolism of particular foods in the diet.

LIST OF SOME HIGH ALKALINE FOODS:
Spinach, molasses, celery, dried figs, carrots, chard, beans, watercress, lettuce, cabbage, broccoli, beets, brussels sprouts, cucumber, parsnips, radish, peas, mushrooms, cauliflower, pineapple, avocado, raisins, dates, melons, cherries, tangerines, strawberries, potatoes, apricots.

LIST OF SOME HIGH ACID FOODS:
Offal, scallops, oysters, lentils, sausage, sardines, beef, lobster, peanuts, haddock, cod, chicken, tuna, salmon, turkey, veal, lamb, whole wheat flour, bacon, eggs, pork, sugar.

CHAPTER SIX

Healing the Gut:
The Four Point Recovery Plan

'The Physician treats but nature heals.'
Hippocrates 460 BC

REMOVE – REPLACE – REPAIR – RESTORE

This is your plan for recovery from symptoms and restoration of health. The following information and advice covers the steps required for you to progress *up the ladder* towards good health, and importantly – what is involved in each step. This knowledge can provide you with the incentive to tackle the task ahead, to persevere and eventually, with gradual improvement, reach your goal.

Medication can give an instant 'quick' fix but this is not a desirable route for restoring health with chronic disease. Nature does not work in this fashion, the healing properties in plants and nutrients work in tune with your body, gently making positive changes, at the same time nourishing and nurturing without causing harm. This is the benefit you derive from natural drug-free healing methods. Healing takes time, and everybody has a different metabolic rate, so patience is the order of the day.

REMOVE

Regardless of the many causative factors of digestive disorders, there are certain steps that need to be applied. All potential gut irritants and allergenic foods should be removed. This following dietary list is specific for healing the gut rather than just addressing the disorder.

DAMAGING FOOD:

It is vital to remove all offending foods and drinks from the diet, to have a 'clean palate' on which to build a new picture of health

- Alcohol, all fizzy and canned drinks, fruit juice (a concentrated sugar form)
- Coffee, black tea, hot chocolate (stimulating beverages)
- Sugar in any form (in ice-cream, biscuits, cakes, most grain products and drinks). Syrups, maple, agave, and honey
- Refined processed foods and white grain products
- Pre-prepared foods with chemical additives
- Red meat and pork (difficult to digest) poorly digested matter can increase risk of bacterial infection
- Polyphosphates in meat and fish, added to increase water content and improve quality[1]
- All bacon, cured and processed cold meats (contain nitrites)
- All dried fruit with sulphites added
- All gluten grains, wheat, rye, barley, oats grown near gluten grain crops

Sulphites are added to wine (some organic wine is sulphite free) and dried fruit as preservatives, nitrites are added to processed and cured meats as preservatives. Both chemical compounds can cause health problems when taken in excess, or when allergic tendencies exist.

UNHEALTHY MICROORGANISMS:

Pathogenic bacteria, yeasts or parasites – where identified with tests, must be eliminated.

There is no rush, and no need to panic if your test results are positive. Your health-care practitioner will be able to advise you on the best steps forward. If you envisage the time it takes to heal safely, avoiding reactions as the body clears out toxins and bugs, every step in the whole picture brings you further forward. As mentioned before, there is no overnight quick 'fix'. Even the act of changing dietary habits can bring untold benefits.

Avoiding offending foods can bring you symptom relief. Once you discover how you can participate in your own healing process, the stress of not knowing what to do or where to turn, is gone. Managing dietary changes is one step that is down to you and your dedication in being strict with yourself.

YOUR FIRST ACTION PLAN:

Is to follow 'The dietary guidelines for a healthy gut' listed in chapter 5 and include 'Super healthy healing foods for the gut' listed below.

Give a few weeks to realise the effect of your initial dietary changes, you may not need to use botanical products at all – healthy prebiotics and probiotics may be sufficient to bring about positive desired changes in health. In some cases dietary changes alone may turn your health around.

It would be best to work in stages, so that you can assess your symptoms in relation to eliminated food items.

YOUR SECOND ACTION PLAN:

If bacterial imbalance is suspected, and here you can refer to my symptoms list in chapter 5 – consider a course of **botanical remedies** listed below. Adhere strictly to manufacturers guidelines on dosage and if you are taking medication or suffer with any diagnosed disease then seek advice from your doctor.

YOUR BEST APPROACH FOR ELIMINATING UNWANTED BUGS

There are thousands of phytochemicals in plants that have inhibitory effects on all types of organisms. It is well recognised that 25–50% of pharmaceutical drugs are derived from plants, but phytotherapy (medicinal plant therapy) is not used in the medical industry as few plants can be licensed as drugs and are therefore non-profitable as antimicrobial agents. Echinacea is the exception to this rule. Never the less – the potency and healing chemicals present in original herbal plants can exceed the healing power of synthetic drugs – and offer treatment that is body compatible.

Researchers in one study, stressed the mounting evidence that many herbs and spices have medicinal properties that can alleviate symptoms or prevent disease.[2]

Using the original plant for therapy is always more beneficial than the synthesised version, as this can never mimic the complete complex healing power of nature from whole, non-isolated plant compounds.

BENEFICIAL BOTANICAL ANTIMICROBIAL AGENTS:

- Grapefruit seed extract
- Garlic
- Oregano
- Clove and cinnamon
- Artemisia
- Goldenseal
- Echinacea
- Berberine, Bearberry
- Black walnut hull

- Pumpkin seed oil
- Pau D'arco

Your body is the most precious thing you own; few people give it the due attention and consideration it deserves. It pays not to overload your body systems with toxins from a poor diet, as the structure of your body that you live in, is your one and only means to a long and healthy life.

Your body will always attempt to recover from wayward habits, but in doing so, you can experience poor health and stress along the way, and you lose valuable worthwhile living time.

REPLACE

SUPER, HEALTHY HEALING FOODS FOR THE GUT

Eating foods which help to increase friendly gut bacteria, is the best way of preventing ill-health. The body has inbuilt mechanisms for keeping us in good health but needs the right fuel to achieve success and build a healthy gut environment.

HEALTHY HEALING FOODS FOR THE GUT:

- Flaxseeds contain both omega 3 and omega 6 oils (useful for individuals who are fish-intolerant). Omega 3 oils have an anti-inflammatory effect and support healthy immune response
- Soaked overnight to produce a mucus like gel, they help protect the gut from irritation and as a cleansing agent help lubricate and move the stools along the intestinal tract
- Walnuts contain omega 3 and 6 oils, providing fibre and healthy fat for the gut. They also protect the heart and help hormonal balance
- Hempseed is very nutritious, rich in calcium and high in protein, it contains no phytic acid, and is ideal as both a fat and protein source for healing the gut
- Organic spirulina, a super food for people suffering with digestive problems, is about 60% easily digestible protein, rich in chlorophyll which aids detoxification, magnesium to help relax

muscles, and is alkaline and full of important trace elements and essential fatty acids

- Light meat, particularly chicken or fish bone broth, rich in collagen, gelatine and protein to help re-build and heal the gut mucosal lining
- Coconut is healing for the gut, it contains saturated fat and caprylic acid which is anti-microbial
- Liquorice has soothing properties to the epithelial tissue lining in the gut, it should be taken in the DGL form which has the glycyrrhizin sweetening content removed, as this can cause potassium loss with regular use
- Onions and garlic are antimicrobial, cleansing and healing and provide sulphur which supports gut health and aids liver detoxification
- Protein whey or casein powder, helps cellular renewal in the gut. It can also help reduce inflammation. Quark contains glutathione, which is supportive of liver detoxification. (These dairy items must be avoided if there is dairy intolerance)
- Kale is vitamin K rich. This vitamin is produced by healthy gut bacteria. If you suffer with increased gut permeability, then deficiency could occur. Include kale in your leafy green intake, also cabbage (particularly savoy – dark green crinkly varieties) which contains vitamin U, and has a soothing, healing effect on the gut tissue, especially for gut ulceration
- Carrots, orange and yellow coloured fruits, provide beta carotene that the body converts to vitamin A, an important nutrient for healing the gut mucosal lining
- Potatoes, raw or cooked contain potassium – are alkaline and soothing on the gut lining
- Sweet potatoes, and root vegetables, a source of prebiotics, help improve bacterial balance in the gut
- Pectin from apples help reduce gut irritation. Cooking them releases the pectin, which also helps bind loose stools
- Sardines, shrimp, tuna, mackerel and other unsmoked oily fish

help provide omega 3 essential fatty acids and vitamin B12 levels which are often affected by malabsorption due to lack of the intrinsic factor in the gut
- Oats and millet contain a lot of silica which is beneficial in skin renewal, improving the integrity of the intestinal lining
- Buttermilk and butter help in gut healing, containing butyric acid, a short chain fatty acid necessary for gut health but obviously to be avoided in dairy intolerance
- Avocados contain vitamin E, potassium, magnesium, essential fatty acids, other nutrients and fibre. Beneficial for antioxidant and nutrient support for the gut
- Wholegrain rice contains gamma oryzanol, a healing agent for the gut
- Carob powder, for cooking and as a drink, contains calcium, many nutrients, lignin a dietary fibre and pectin which soothes the gut, reduces inflammation and improves elimination. It is useful in controlling diarrhoea and digestive upsets. Having a 'chocolatey' flavour, it can be used to replace chocolate

EXTRA LIVER AND INTESTINAL SUPPORT:
- Reduced glutathione, to aid liver metabolism and help excrete bacteria
- Milk thistle, as a gentle liver tonic
- Psyllium husk to increase peristalsis and cleanse the intestines
- Cascara for cleansing with gentle laxative properties

After successfully eliminating damaging, disease causing pathogens, the gut environment has cleansed itself out, cleared up inflammation and, hopefully responded positively to its nutritious healthy diet.

There are numerous studies showing the enormous medicinal benefits from plant derived compounds. Researchers in one study found that "biological and therapeutic properties attributed to these plant metabolites include antioxidant, anti-inflammatory, antimicrobial and anti-cancer activities."[3]

Pandey and Rizvi in their research in 2009, state that, after absorption, the phytochemicals in plants go to support liver detoxification pathways. Plants have many properties as well as antioxidant benefits, they also play a role in supporting sulphation, methylation and glucuronidation detoxification pathways in the liver.

This study concludes that consuming a diet rich in antioxidants, has been associated with reduced levels of oxidative damage to DNA.[4]

Including a wide range of plant foods in your diet can benefit every system. There are thousands of phytochemicals in food that supply medicine for the body, it is just a question of recognising what nature has on offer.

Supplementation with – digestive herbs, dandelion, globe artichoke (bitters, which stimulate the production of bile) plant digestive enzymes, pepsin, and betaine hydrochloride, will help address deficiencies in digestive enzymes and stomach acid. All these measures will encourage better digestion.

Care must be taken using digestive enzymes and HCL (hydrochloride) when inflammation or irritation exists in the gut. You must wait until the inflammation is under control. Plant based enzymes are very gentle; I do not recommend animal-based enzymes or ox bile supplements, their potency can contribute to intestinal erosion in the human body.

REPAIR

NUTRIENTS AND HEALING AGENTS FOR THE GUT MUCOSA:

- **Essential fatty acids, GLA, EPA, DHA**

Fatty acids are natural components of fats and oils. Most can be synthesised by the body with essential fats from the diet, but omega 3 and 6 fatty acids are called essential as the body cannot produce them and additionally cannot do without them; they are vital to health in the human body.

Essential fatty acids such as GLA, gamma linolenic acid, DHA, docosahexaenoic acid and EPA, eicosapentaenoic acid, need to be supplied in the diet.

These unsaturated fatty acids are required for hormone balance, skin lubrication, neurological function, cardiovascular health, proper growth in childhood and for structure and maintenance of all cell membranes. They also exert an anti-inflammatory effect.

This latter role is where the omega oils come into play, to reduce inflammation and help maintain intestinal gut lining integrity. Polyunsaturated fatty acids GLA, EPA and DHA have been found to help heal a leaky gut and improve gut barrier function.[5]

Omega 3 and 6 oils come from oily fish, nuts, seeds, soya beans and green leafy vegetables. They are converted by enzyme activity – in the body to an active form called prostaglandins – a hormone type of substance with both inflammatory and anti-inflammatory action.

Uncontrolled inflammation can develop with a high meat-based diet lacking in omega oils. Omega 3 oils have been shown in recent studies to reduce inflammation and restore mucosal permeability in the gut.[6]

Omega 3 and omega 6 oils are incorporated into membrane phospholipids in mucosal epithelial cells and exert a healing action.

Uncontrolled inflammatory conditions can also occur when the diet is low in omega 3 fatty acids from oily fish, walnuts and flaxseeds and imbalanced with excessive omega 6 intake from processed stabilised cooking oils. The typical western diet is higher in omega 6 fatty acids than omega 3. The higher the level of omega 3 oils from oily fish, walnuts and linseeds in your diet, the more control you will have over inflammatory processes.

Prostaglandins have many other roles in body activity but, we will focus on digestive support. They regulate the gut smooth muscle action and support protective mucosal secretions.

Deficiencies of prostaglandins can lead to a loss of protection in the mucosal lining and hinder the healing process.

FACTORS THAT REDUCE FATTY ACID CONVERSION TO PROSTAGLANDINS:

- Chronic stress
- Ageing
- Excessive caffeine intake
- Alcohol intake, smoking
- Nutritional deficiencies
- Trans fats (hydrogenated, processed cooking fats and oils). These act like saturated fats, due to molecular structure damage
- Burnt barbecued foods

The conversion by enzymes is dependent on the nutrients – vitamin C, vitamins B3 and 6, biotin, zinc and magnesium.

- **L-Glutamine,** to nourish the cells in the epithelial lining. L-Glutamine and Glucosamine are the most recognised aids to healing the gut.[6] Glucosamine is what is known as a pre-cursor (the raw material) for mucosal glycoproteins, the mucous coating which protects the cells in the gut wall

L-Glutamine is the primary nutrient for the gut, this important amino acid provides fuel for the brain, immune system and feeds cells that line the intestinal tract, helping to maintain integrity of the mucosal lining and improving gut permeability. Proper functioning and regulation of tight junctions in the gut is crucial. One study in 2010 stated that "Glutamine is the best-known compound for reducing intestinal permeability and nutritional depletion is known to result in increased intestinal permeability".[7]

Glutamine is available from the diet in such foods as meat, fish, eggs, dairy and plant foods but cooking can easily reduce its availability.

- **LRT, Lipid replacement therapy.** Healthy lipids (glycophospholipids) are fats required for building healthy cell membranes and repairing damaged intestinal tissue. There is interesting anecdotal feedback concerning Lipid Replacement Therapy, using isolated glycophospholipids derived from food. Consistent benefits were seen in improved energy and pain for fatigued and arthritic patients and increased endothelial cell renewal in gut disorders. Because of the rapid turnover in gut cell renewal, lipids can play a considerable role in the re-building of healthy cell membranes[8]

Phospholipids a major component of cell membranes, are found in egg yolk as lecithin and in many plants – soya, sunflower and rapeseeds. Soya should not be GM. Gene manipulated foods are highly suspect in damaging human health, the human body does not contain enzymes that can recognise and metabolise such foreign material. Clinical trials have shown the benefits of LRT in restoring and maintaining membrane function by the nature of replacing damaged membrane phospholipids.[9]

- Zinc, vitamins A, E, and C, B5, B6, help cellular repair and tissue renewal
- **N.A.G. (N-Acetyl Glucosamine),** heals connective tissue in the gut. NAG consists of an amino acid and glucose, called an amino sugar. This supplies support, together with protein for building structure in cell membranes, an essential component of body tissues, helping to hold cells together
- **MSM, (methyl sulphonyl methane)** from sulphur containing foods, protect against excessive cell oxidation
- **Gamma oryzanol,** soothes the mucosal lining and helps maintain gastric secretion
- **Marshmallow,** a source of mucilage that soothes, protects and reduces irritation

- **Slippery elm,** a buffer on epithelial tissue, protecting against irritation from food

There are many nutritional healing aids in food, nature's medicine chest, and supplements derived from food bases, work extremely well in helping reverse distressing symptoms experienced with digestive disorders.

Many studies on the effects of nutritional support have found that certain nutritional factors may help support mucosal health and promote normal intestinal permeability. These factors include antioxidant and mucosal nutrients, digestive enzymes and fibre.[10]

Amino acids and healthy fats are required for the building structure of cells, which contain protein and fat in the structure of the cell membrane. For gut healing measures, a higher level of complete protein should be eaten, but always combined with healthy portions of fruit and vegetables, for healthy bowel function. The protein should be 'light' – eggs, fish, chicken or lamb.

ADDING LACTO-FERMENTED FOODS

Foods which have been cultured or fermented with bacteria, produce lactic acid, which stops the food from spoiling. This was the method of preserving food over centuries and is still practiced in indigenous tribes who live in hot countries and have no access to refrigerators.

Lactic acid containing foods help heal the gut, detract pathogens, provide healthy enzymes and can help to restore gut health by balancing acid alkaline levels. Fermented vegetables have a higher level of nutrients and should be included where possible in the diet. Liquid whey containing lactic acid is also beneficial.

Some individuals do not tolerate fermented foods, due to the acidic nature of the produce, but one or two varieties may be added gradually, combined with other foods. Food tolerance varies with the time of day as the body phases through metabolic functions; it is worthwhile experimenting with a change in timing of fermented food intake.

LACTO-FERMENTED FOOD LIST:

- Sauerkraut
- Yoghurt
- Pickles
- Raw cheese
- Kefir
- Kombucha
- Miso
- Tempeh
- Natto, fermented soy (only GMO-free)
- Kimchi

ADDING ANTIOXIDANTS

These elements support the immune system by protecting the body cells from harmful molecules called free radicals. Free radical damage in cells occurs in normal every-day metabolism but the body has inbuilt enzyme systems that mop up the damage. A regular intake of protective antioxidants in our food supply is necessary, to supply raw materials for these enzymes to work efficiently. Vitamins A, C, E and selenium and zinc are nutrient antioxidants, together with fruit and vegetable coloured pigments, called phytochemicals. Eating your way through the rainbow should be your aim at every meal.

ANTIOXIDANTS, PHYTOCHEMICALS IN FOOD, HERBS AND SPICES:

- Lycopene, the red pigment in tomatoes, berries and other foods
- Lutein, the yellow pigment in yellow peppers and fruits and vegetables
- Carotenoid, beta carotene, the yellow-orange pigments in carrots, mango and other fruits

- Anthocyanins, the red, purple, blue, black pigments in berries and black rice and beans
- Chlorophyll, the green pigment in dark green leafy vegetables, which also contains magnesium

Antioxidant and other bioactive properties exist in many spices and herbs including:

Cloves, ginger, peppermint, allspice, aniseeds, saffron, sage, rosemary, thyme, cumin, cinnamon, oregano, grapeseed extract and green tea.

Hesperidin, lipoic acid, quercetin, curcumin, pine bark extract and reduced glutathione are some beneficial bioactive compounds and chemicals which help to keep the body healthy.

These food items have medicinal properties, help to reduce inflammation, fight infection and protect cells from DNA damage.

RESTORE

ADDING PROBIOTICS:

Lactobacillus species which reside mostly in the small intestines and Bifidobacterium which live in the large bowel.

There are trillions of species of bacteria that reside in our gut, most of which are 'friendly' and supporting health. They prevent invasion from opportunistic pathogenic bacteria, help to regulate cholesterol, produce B vitamins, vitamin K and help regulate the immune system.

All effort should be made to keep them happily multiplying.

Probiotics are micro-organisms, specially cultured friendly bacteria that are beneficial for restoring health in the gastrointestinal tract. For healing a damaged compromised gut, therapy with probiotics has been shown to be therapeutic in reducing symptoms of IBS.[11]

FACTORS THAT AFFECT YOUR LEVEL OF FRIENDLY BACTERIA:

- Antibiotic use
- Low fibre diet
- Contaminated food and water
- Travel in foreign countries
- Medication and social drugs
- Low calorie poorly balanced diet.
- Alcohol consumption, smoking
- Stressful lifestyle

When digestive disorders exist, there is also evidence of dysbiosis (imbalanced gut bacteria). Supplementation is useful for individuals with disturbed bacterial flora, supplying extra micro-organisms to help re-establish a healthy microflora. The diet should then contain prebiotics in beneficial fibre rich foods, to provide food for healthy colonisation of these organisms.

ADDING PREBIOTICS:

Prebiotics act as food for probiotics, stimulating growth of beneficial or friendly bacteria such as Lactobacilli and Bifidobacterium species, which increase resistance to pathogens, and helps you to remain in good health.

- It is important the diet contains these essential 'growth' factors. Humans can't digest fibre-rich material, but it is the perfect food for gut bacteria. Inulin fibre is the most common prebiotic found in the following foods:
- **Garlic, onions, leeks, Jerusalem artichoke, chicory bananas, oats and seaweed, asparagus, flaxseeds, apples, celery**

Many foods including the above, contain a natural source of prebiotic fibre called **Fructo-oligosaccharide or FOS** that is beneficial in generating growth factors for the bacteria which reside in the small and large bowel. It also aids mineral absorption. It can be used as a bulking agent to help improve peristalsis in the intestinal tract, but caution should be applied in dose levels used, or it may cause or increase bloating.

FOS is fermented by Bifidobacterium in the colon producing short chain fatty acids, acetate, lactate, butyrate and propionate, that keep the gut and body healthy. Half of the weight of your stools are composed by bacteria.

The more diverse the species, the greater the benefit in intestinal health. Many clinical trials have indicated the benefits derived from probiotic supplementation. One study found a significant reduction in IBS symptoms when a multi strain probiotic was given.[12]

Replacing healthy friendly bacteria by supplementation with broad spectrum probiotics is recommended. Broad spectrum means a broad variety of strains and species to achieve diversity in the microflora, your potential colony of healthy microbes.

There are many on the market, but always aim for strains with a variety of Lactobacillus acidophilus and Bifidobacterium, the two most prolific organisms in the intestinal tract, that can survive in the presence of bile and stomach acid and will adhere to the intestinal wall.

In the case of probiotics, usually cheaper brands provide less health benefits.

There are probiotic supplements available both human-based and soil-based, it would be best to seek practitioner advice on appropriate strains, strengths and origins, should you be suffering with debilitating digestive disease, and require specialised probiotic support.

THE ROLE OF FIBRE IN MAINTAINNG HEALTHY GUT FLORA

Healthy stools in colour and consistency are an indication all is well in your gut. The food material you eat forms the stools, the amount and type of liquid you drink regulates the fluid balance within the stools and the healthy passageway of the waste material throughout the intestinal tract.

FUNCTIONS OF FIBRE:

- Absorbs water, helping to provide a gel-type mass which improves stool formation
- Increases stool bulk
- Both increases and decreases transit time of stools through digestive tract, vital in dealing with constipation and diarrhoea
- Facilitates healthy bacterial balance by providing food for bacteria to ferment
- Help regulate cholesterol levels and improve cardiovascular health
- Slows the rate sugar absorbed into the bloodstream, helping blood sugar balance
- Maintains healthy function of the peristaltic movement in the intestinal tract
- Helps to cleanse and detoxify the body by removing toxins from the gut

There are many foods containing fibre, but it is the balance you take in that is important. The human body functions best on an intake of both soluble and insoluble fibre. Regular intake of water is required when you increase your fibre intake, otherwise you may find stools are difficult to pass.

Fruit and vegetables contain both types of fibre. It is best, rather than getting stressed trying to include both types, for you to focus on a varied diet of fruit, vegetables, grains, nuts, seeds and legumes.

SOLUBLE FIBRE – absorbs water and produces a gel.

Beans, peas, lentils, oats, barley, nuts and seeds and psyllium a fibre supplement, also found in certain fruit and vegetables.

INSOLUBLE FIBRE – does not absorb water but remains in the gut in the same form.

The outer husk in wholegrains, some fruit and vegetables such as celery, the outer husk in seeds or beans and peas and some skins on food.

CHAPTER SEVEN

Detoxification: Liver Support

'May the inward and outward man be as one.'
Socrates 469 BC

WHY IS IT ESSENTIAL TO SUPPORT THE LIVER WHILST HEALING THE GUT?

Over your lifetime, you are exposed to many foreign chemicals, even if you eat a super organic diet and avoid food additives. It is inevitable in this toxic world we all live in.

Chemical exposure affects your body. Chemicals are present in the food you eat, pesticide and herbicide residues commonly found in random food checks; the water you drink, the air you breathe, from plastic food packaging, from thousands of damaging toxic compounds in body care products, drugs and from synthetic hormones in the contraceptive pill or HRT.

If your body is not 'clean from within' and the liver is struggling to detoxify all these harmful compounds, then the treatment of digestive disorders will take longer to resolve, as toxins hinder healthy digestive function.

For protection, limit exposure where possible and eat a diet rich in supporting nutrients that help the body detoxify these damaging substances. The body's ability to rid itself of toxic substances is largely dependent on the liver. Scientific research has revealed several compounds in plant foods, that help support the liver detoxification processes that deal with the metabolism of damaging toxic substances.[1]

> *'In all things of nature, there is something of the marvellous.'*
> Aristotle 384 BC

ENTER THE LIVER AND THE P450 ENZYME SYSTEM

The liver is the most important organ for keeping your body healthy. It changes or detoxifies harmful substances, converting them by enzyme activity, into water-soluble forms that the body can safely excrete via the kidneys and bowels.

This whole metabolic process, is referred to as biotransformation. The removal of drugs and hormones takes place by chemically altering them in preparation for the process of excretion.

The cytochrome P450 liver enzymes are essential for metabolising drugs, hormones and toxins that either enter the body from external sources or come from within the body systems.

The enzyme activity is dependent on vitamins and minerals that come from your diet, specifically B vitamins, magnesium, zinc, vitamin A, selenium, vitamin C and vitamin E, copper and amino acids from protein.

The liver uses two mechanisms – phase 1 and phase 2, to remove toxins with the help of the powerful cytochrome P450 enzyme system. These enzymes are found in a high concentration in the liver, working to metabolise potential toxic compounds into a form that is safe for the body to excrete.

THE PROCESS OF DETOXIFICATION AND ELIMINATION

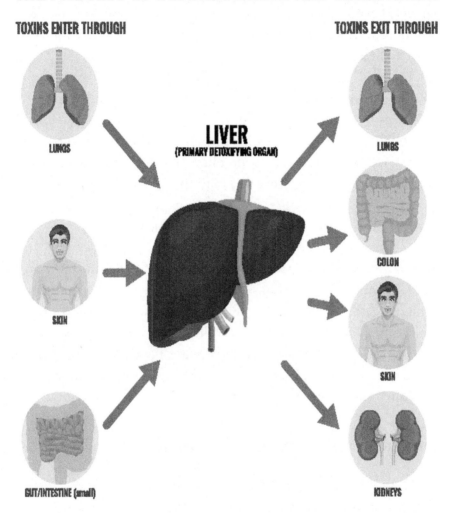

Toxic waste in your body can originate from: food additives, pesticides, herbicides, airborne pollutants, medication, tobacco, drugs, dental materials, household and bodycare chemicals and microbial infection from faulty digestion.

In a scientific review in 2015 investigating the influence of food components on metabolic detoxification pathways, researchers stated that for phase 1 and phase 2 mechanisms, clinical recommendations with food-derived components, help to reduce the negative impact of toxins and enhance phase 1 and 2 pathways.[2]

PHASE 1: involves your body's own enzyme systems activating toxic substances to make them accessible to phase 2 enzyme mechanisms. This involves neutralising free radicals with the use of nutritional and dietary antioxidants – red, blue, black, purple pigments in fruit, an antioxidant rich diet and glutathione rich foods – avocado, asparagus, melon, walnuts, garlic, onions and cruciferous greens. The herb milk thistle is beneficial in this phase.

PHASE 2: converts the partially metabolised toxins, into a water-soluble form for excretion. This is achieved with conjugation (joining together) with certain amino acids from protein in your diet. Your body then eliminates them via the kidneys and bowels in urine and stools. Foods that aid this process are found in a high protein diet, garlic, onions, leeks, brussels sprouts, cauliflower, citrus fruits (excluding grapefruit) and whey powder.

DETOXIFICATION FUNCTIONS BY THE LIVER:

- Metabolises, filters and eliminates wastes
- Neutralises toxins and carcinogenic substances
- Reduces auto-toxification, and re-cycling of toxic substances
- Ensures a good production and flow of bile, to enhance toxin excretion
- Metabolises substances that stagnate, putrefy and ferment
- Facilitates toxin elimination via skin, lungs, kidneys, bowels

ARE YOU A POOR DETOXIFIER?

These two pathways can sometimes be imbalanced in certain individuals. This may be due to dysbiosis in the gut (an imbalance in gut bacteria), nutritional deficiencies, chronic stress, overload of toxins, poor liver function, poor elimination, dehydration, lack of exercise, poor circulation, or simply by the process of ageing.

Phase 1 or 2 may be under or over functioning, or there may be disharmony within the two phases. Overall, this can cause poor detoxification.

If your body's detoxification ability is under functioning, there is a danger that harmful substances are recycled in the body via the blood stream, potentially contributing to symptoms of poor health, headaches, muscle and joint pain, skin complaints, mental health problems, hormonal and digestive disturbances.

These toxins can migrate to the brain and central nervous system cells, causing further health problems.

Chronic constipation is an issue, this is sometimes referred to as a toxic bowel, where stagnant waste material in the intestinal tract, can get re-absorbed, causing yet more overload to body elimination processes.

The toxins that the body is confronted with, from external pollution, dietary intake, medication, alcohol and environmental sources are called exotoxins.

Endotoxins are produced within the body from normal metabolic processes; producing various acids, urea, bilirubin and ammonia, together with toxins produced by unfriendly intestinal bacteria.

All these harmful substances need metabolising and excreting. The less time they spend in the body – the better.

SIGNS OF POOR LIVER FUNCTION:

- Dark circles, puffiness and bags under the eyes
- Yellow tinge to whites of eyes
- Itchy skin

- Headaches, mood swings, poor concentration
- Fluid retention
- Constipation

THE EFFECTS OF POOR DETOXIFICATION:

- Increased infections, poor immune function
- Tissue damage and increased degeneration of cells
- Hormonal disturbances
- Food intolerance, allergies and leaky gut syndrome
- Digestive diseases, inflammatory bowel disease
- Mental health problems
- Autoimmune disease
- Skin conditions
- Gall bladder problems
- Chronic fatigue

According to the Canadian Liver Foundation:

The liver is the most metabolically complex organ in the entire body; performing over 500 different metabolic functions, fighting off infection, neutralising toxins, manufacturing protein and hormones, controlling blood sugar and helping blood clotting. These are just some of the functions that are recognised and understood by scientists.

The liver also stores fat soluble vitamins, A, D E, K, also vitamin B12, some vitamin C and the minerals iron and copper. Worn-out red blood cells are metabolised in the liver, resulting in bilirubin formation. Bilirubin is the yellow-brown pigment seen in bile, it deodorises the stools and helps intestinal function in digestive processes. Bile contains no digestive enzymes and consists mostly of water, bile salts and bile pigments. Every day the liver produces approximately 800–1,000 milligrams of bile.

The function of bile, which is produced in the liver and stored in the gallbladder, is for the emulsification of fats in the diet, it helps to break them down into small fractions called micelles, which are in an easier form for absorption. When dietary fats or lipids as they are known, are not well absorbed, as in the case after surgery for removal of the gallbladder, then fat soluble vitamins A, D, E, and K absorption can be reduced.

The main nutrients that support liver function are vitamins A, D, E, K, B complex, choline, inositol, vitamin C, and the minerals iron, copper, selenium, magnesium, and potassium. Amino acids from dietary protein intake are also vital for detoxification function.

The branched chain amino acids; leucine, glycine, isoleucine, valine and taurine plus cysteine are involved in conjugation function, namely the binding of toxic substances to amino acids for the process of metabolising and excreting. Therefore, a high protein diet is recommended for treating digestive disorders.

Glutathione is the most important antioxidant found in every cell of the body. It is naturally produced in the body and consists of three amino acids – cysteine, glutamic acid and glycine, which help repair damaged cells.

Levels reduce with ageing, disease, oxidative stress, free radical cell damage, high alcohol intake, enzyme deficiency, and nutritional deficiencies, particularly vitamin C and E. This antioxidant is essential for healthy liver function.

FOODS THAT STIMULATE GLUTATHIONE PRODUCTION

Cruciferous vegetables:
- Cabbage, kale, Brussels sprouts, broccoli, radish, turnips, watercress, arugula salad, kohlrabi and chard.
- All green leafy vegetables and colourful fruits and berries, salads, greens and vegetables offer support as antioxidants and help to stimulate glutathione activity.
- Whey powder, green tea, selenium rich foods, brazil nuts, mushrooms, fish, brown rice, seeds and greens. The herb milk thistle.

SULPHUR RICH FOODS FOR LIVER SUPPORT:

Sulphur, from dietary intake of cruciferous vegetables, onions, garlic, horseradish, mustard, cauliflower and eggs provides support for liver detoxification; nutrients are utilised to convert steroid hormones, drugs, alcohol, and other substances of endogenous origin into a form safe for excretion.

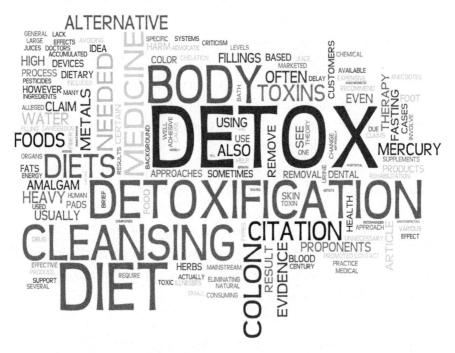

**WHAT YOU SHOULD INCLUDE
IN YOUR DIET FOR LIVER SUPPORT:**

*   Beetroot, olive oil, carrots, dandelion, globe artichoke, fennel, chicory and citrus fruit
*   Herbs and spices: ginger, golden rod, kelp, curcumin, holy basil, horsetail and knotgrass

The above listed foods can help flush out toxins, stimulate bile flow and improve liver function.

Research discussion in 2011 published in the *Journal of Alternative and Complementary Medicine*, pointed out that "As increasing evidence of the relationship between body burden, and adverse effects of synthetic chemicals emerge; safe and effective methods of reducing this load as used with naturopathic doctors, may serve as an adequate means to reduce the body burden of synthetic chemicals found today in humans."[3]

AROMATIC ESSENTIAL OILS

> *'The way to health is to have an aromatic bath and a scented massage each day.'*
> Hippocrates 460 BC

Essential oils are highly volatile fragrances in herbs and flowers, they are extracted by distillation and can evaporate readily.

There are many healthy properties in all essential oils, some oils have antibacterial and antifungal properties, others have calming, relaxing effects that help to reduce stress and anxiety. Rosemary for instance, has stimulating properties, helps the circulation and can aid lymph drainage which helps clear waste products from the body – so important in the detoxification process. Lavender oil rubbed on the body before sleep has wonderful relaxing properties, it is also antibacterial, antiseptic and has wound healing properties. A few drops in your bath can relieve stress and relax the body.

According to Robert Tisserand, a leading figure in the field of aromatherapy and Editor of the *International Journal of Aromatherapy*, "aromatherapy is of considerable help for common stress-related and minor disorders" including such conditions as moderate anxiety, depression and digestive disorders.[4]

He writes of potions of volatile herbs recommended in the 1600s as protection against the plague: including cloves, juniper, nutmeg, rue, rosemary, sage, mastic, incense, myrtle, musk, elder and wormwood. Many of these herbs are recognised today for their potent properties for warding off infection and use as anti-parasitic agents. Aromatic oils are absorbed rapidly through the skin and into cells.

To enhance your gut healing and detoxification programme, I would recommend finding a proficient practitioner who can recommend a supportive programme to help relaxation and stress.

HYDROTHERAPY

Water has endless healing potential and can be applied in many ways to induce the body to detoxify and relax, and to improve health and vitality. If you feel calm, comfortable and in control and can relieve stress with a warm bath or shower, then your relaxed nervous system will influence your digestive processes.

Leon Chaitow mentions in his book *Hydrotherapy* that it is possible to de-activate many viruses and bacteria by heating the body temperature using water, as these organisms are heat sensitive.[5]

Fevers are the immune system's defence mechanism against pathogen attack. A similar less potent effect may be achieved by a warm bath, an emersion in body temperature bath water, with some drops of antimicrobial essential oils.

For supporting detoxification, a simple bath with Epsom salts, sea-salt or algae seaweed, can open the pores, relax the muscles, alkalise the body and aid elimination. Before bathing, dry skin brushing can stimulate the skin surface and help the elimination of toxins through skin pores.

Foot baths with essential oils can help circulation, immune function and relaxation.

Saunas: widely popular, are not, however for everyone. Valuable minerals and trace elements are lost in sweating, these nutrients need replacing. Individuals with imbalanced electrolytes (sodium and potassium levels) and health problems with hypo or hypertension should avoid saunas as they can promote faintness or dizzy spells.

EXERCISE, LIGHT AND SUNLIGHT

If you are not a fan of going to the gym, there are many choices of exercise available and surely something that can appeal to you. Outdoor exercise is always healthier than indoor activities.

The human body is designed to thrive on movement and sunshine. If uninspired to exercise communally, a daily brisk walk is a must. A daily sun dose is required for our vitamin D levels, which occur when bare skin is exposed to sunlight (not over midday). Even when the sun is not shining, light is important, it hits the rods in the eye and helps maintain vital vitamin A levels.

With attention paid to your new dietary regime, the techniques and tips highlighted above, you should be well on the way to achieving good health.

CHAPTER EIGHT

Mindful Shopping and Eating for Health and Pleasure

'The greatest medicine of all is teaching people how not to need it.'
Hippocrates 460 BC

Food, and only food is your healing power for maintaining good health. Supplements and super food or botanical concentrates that provide therapeutic value, are not to be used in the place of a healthy diet, for the main reason that all the phytochemical extracts that have healing properties require nutrients from a well-balanced dietary intake to be well absorbed. They supplement and complement your diet, but do not replace it.

Nutrients in any form do not work in isolation in the human body, they work synergistically as 'co-factors'. Vitamins work together with minerals in any number of combinations; amino acids, fatty acids require vitamins and minerals for digestion and absorption. Some vitamins, vitamin A, D, E and K are fat soluble and need lipids, fats or oils in the diet for absorption. There are dozens of nutrients we require daily to keep fit and healthy.

You can, with determined effort, eat yourself well again. It need not be an expensive exercise, but you do need to have the knowledge to know what nutrients the body requires, and not only that, to understand how food manufacturing processes can destroy the very nutrients you think you are buying in your shopping sprees. That is money down the drain; this requires what I call mindful shopping, just being aware and to read labels carefully.

QUALITY NOT QUANTITY

You can quite purposely ignore all the marketing hype and advertising designed to encourage people to buy certain products in shops, and home in on your section in the shop – of healthy organic additive-free foods being safe in the knowledge that you have identified to the best of your knowledge, the most nutritious options available in this confusing world of processed foods and excess food supply.

Manufacturing giants who are trying to feed nations with cheap sub-quality produce, devoid of all the precious nutrients nature provides, should be deterred. Once healthy food is identified, avoid temptation and learn how to recognise the real benefits gained in real food as opposed to the ill effects expected from the junk food option.

How many of us love shopping for food? For most it is only a necessary chore.

There are many benefits to be had in focused shopping. Gaining extra time in your life, avoiding the frenetic mad weekend or holiday scrum to stock up with trolley loads of fast food. This focused way of shopping can help relieve the stress of even considering the enormous magnitude and mammoth variety of processed foods offered by the supermarkets.

The human body requires very little in the way of calories, in relation to the vast amounts on offer. The single most important fact to consider, is that fewer calories and more nutrients within the calories is the healthiest way of eating. It is probably not the best idea to go food shopping whilst hungry or having missed a meal, as more food is piled in the trolleys than the body needs.

The trick is to remain neutral to all the food choices on offer unless you have identified healthy options. Read labels (if you don't recognise the ingredient as food, it is possibly a nasty additive).

The choices available can be varied and wide within these main categories – organic, local naturally reared produce, unprocessed, sugar- and additive-free products in their whole, nutrient-rich forms.

Organically traditionally grown produce is far superior to non-organic alternatives. Levels of vitamins, minerals, trace elements and plant chemicals are higher in unsprayed produce and the robust structure of organic plants withstand attack by insects or disease, far better than the weakened often hybrid versions of food grown with conventional farming. Once you start to eat nutrient rich unprocessed foods, you will start to feel the benefits; increased energy levels, healthy nails, skin and hair, improved sleeping patterns, and above all improved digestive health.

EAT ORGANIC FOR GOODNESS' SAKE

Supporting organic farmers contributes to welfare of the soil, humans and the planet.

Professor P. Grandjean, adjunct Professor of Environmental Health in the US, outlines in his report, the health benefits of eating organic food and practising organic agriculture.[1]

It may be more expensive but other savings can be made when shopping for real food as nature provides. Savings can be made through having less choice of ready-made processed produce, what is generally termed 'junk food', manipulated and manufactured by man. The main advantage in buying only organic produce is the huge benefit to health, which cannot be measured in terms of cost.

Recent research in both 2015 and 2016, in a total of over 343 studies, by a team led by Professor Leifert from Newcastle University, involved the most extensive analysis of nutrient content in organic food, ever undertaken.

The evidence shown was overwhelming in favour of organic crops. These contained 50% lower levels of toxic heavy metals, 50% more omega fatty acids in dairy and meat, and 60% higher levels of antioxidants in fruit and vegetables. The conclusion reached, was that there was a growing body of documented evidence to demonstrate just how profoundly farming methods can influence nutritional content of food.[2,3]

Which produce would you prefer to eat; chemically laden toxic food or nutrient-rich healthy food? There really should not be any discussion over this issue, if you value what you put into your body.

To make up for the nutrient deficit created by modern agriculture farming practices, manufacturers will often add in synthetic nutrients. As the body only recognises mother nature's natural unadulterated nutrients, synthetic versions can quickly add to the body's toxic load.

EAT YOURSELF HEALTHY

Nothing should be presumed to be 100% healthy, even with organic produce, you may note as an example that sugar is added in organic jams or other organic produce. High fructose corn syrup, sucrose, fructose, are all extremely damaging to health. They are manipulated processed sugars that damage body tissues.

Taking steps to source sugar-free organic foods is the only way forward as the extra cost for the 'organic label' is short changing you in health. Shop around as there are alternatives to the large commercial companies, who jump on the organic 'bandwagon' for profit.

There are many small reputable dedicated companies that go to extremes, in ensuring your organic food is sugar- and additive-free and as healthy as possible – these need your support. Check farmers' markets, online businesses and home-made produce locally, even without the 'organic' label certification, which is expensive to buy. Many smaller firms are pesticide, herbicide and chemical free, and obviously can sell at more affordable prices.

Supermarket organic produce may sit under light and heat or be exposed to chilled temperatures, all detrimental to the nutrient content. Encased in plastic – it is hardly the health product you should be seeking.

Artificial sweeteners, such as cyclamate, aspartame, sucralose, acesulfame potassium (K) and saccharin should be completely avoided, they are toxic substances, that the body cannot recognise and therefore can be metabolised in the body to other dangerous chemical compounds that can have carcinogenic properties.

THE QUESTION OF DAIRY

Many people do not have a problem tolerating dairy but with the process of homogenisation and pasteurisation, nutrients such as calcium become less available, and protein can become less soluble. Dairy is not to be relied upon as a major source of nutrients, that fact applies to calves, not humans.

Raw dairy products contain higher levels of nutrients but pose a risk through potential microbial infection. If you can find raw unpasteurised cheese, this would be more nutritious. In the process of cheese making the risk of infection diminishes, though in soft cheese it can remain a risk. Raw unpasteurised yoghurt, which has the lactose (milk sugar) converted to lactic acid in the fermentation process has anti-microbial effects and can provide some health benefits.

Dairy intolerant individuals can react to lactose or the protein content of milk (casein). By conversion to yoghurt or cheese the lactose has been altered chemically. It is sometimes possible to tolerate these dairy forms but not taken as milk.

As an alternative to cow's dairy, goat's milk products are more easily tolerated, being lower in protein and lighter to digest. It is quite possible, however to be dairy free and healthy, this choice is down to the individual.

When suffering with digestive problems, dairy should be avoided, until a positive outcome from dietary changes and therapeutic treatment is seen. Dairy products offer more choice in the diet but for some individuals it puts added stress on digestive processes.

A recent animal research article, found that food allergy and anaphylactic shock occurred in feeding animals pasteurised milk proteins. Pasteurisation caused aggregation of milk protein and this can inhibit uptake by epithelial cells.[4]

Another side of the picture has been seen in a review of 52 clinical trials on dairy produce and inflammation. The conclusion suggests that dairy produce that has been fermented can provide anti-inflammatory properties in humans, who are not suffering with milk allergy.[5]

With the right timing, you may find fermented dairy items can help improve your digestive problems, but caution should be applied.

AVOID GM FOODS

These foods mainly found in corn, alfalfa, squash, zucchini, soya, canola, sugar beet, but is increasingly being applied to other foods, are unbelievably threatening to mankind: man manipulated freakish poor substitutes for the real food item, but capable of making huge profits for Monsanto, the company behind the products. Contamination of food crops with damaging foreign gene species is a threat throughout the world. These foods are fed to animals in the USA to reduce the need for pasture feeding, so are getting through the food chain into humans from milk and meat consumption.

GM foods have been exposed to the herbicide Roundup which contains glyphosate. This herbicide was specifically developed to be used in the GM industry as the genetically manipulated foods are produced to tolerate the toxic effect when crops are sprayed to kill weeds.

These foods, which since being marketed around the world as an excuse for feeding the multitudes, have resulted in foetal malformation, low sperm count in males and signs of ill health in people working with the pesticide in many countries and presents one of the biggest health threats in our food chain world-wide, should progress in development be allowed to continue.

The suspected impact on gastrointestinal health has been profound. These unhealthy manipulated foods and the toxic residues of Roundup found in their structure, have been implicated in increased incidence world-wide in gut permeability, allergies, food intolerance, immune and auto-immune disease, damage to the intestinal wall and digestive disorders.[6]

AVOID FOOD LADEN WITH PESTICIDES

The more the body is over laden with chemicals and toxins the harder it needs to work to keep you healthy. Modern farming agriculture practices are swamping the land with noxious, toxic chemicals.

This has steadily increased since the Second World War and more and more chemicals, some banned in certain countries, are found to be causing enormous health risks to humans. Over the years I have treated people with allergic reactions from environmental chemicals, which were linked to living close by conventionally sprayed orchards and fields. Numerous research studies show evidence of health issues arising from toxic sprays on our food supply.[7]

BE HEALTHY INSIDE-OUT

There are potentially very harmful ingredients in personal care products, from heavy metals, sodium lauryl sulphate, mineral oils, formaldehyde, fluorocarbons and other body damaging chemicals. All these artificial chemicals, in lotions, bath products, shampoos, toothpaste even, though not eaten, will be absorbed through the skin and cause a toxic burden on the liver. The plastic packaging is another polluting issue.

REDUCING OXALATES AND PHYTATES

All plants contain compounds that help detract insects and protect them from attack. These plant toxins have only a minor effect on humans but they can act to interfere with nutrient absorption and inhibit our body enzyme systems which in turn can lead to reduced digestive function.

It is wise to reduce intake of oxalate-rich foods, just eating them occasionally. Oxalic acid found in significant levels in rhubarb and spinach, interferes with calcium absorption, by binding with calcium to produce calcium oxalate, which can in turn increase risk of kidney stones.

Phytic acid (the storage form of phosphorus) found in the outer husk of wholegrains, beans, seeds and pulses, binds to minerals in the gut. These substances interfere with digestion, and chelate (bind) with calcium, zinc and iron, reducing absorption of these vital minerals in the gastrointestinal tract. One positive fact emerged in one research article: phytic acid had been found to form a unique chelate with iron allowing it to act as a powerful antioxidant suppressing oxidative reactions.[8]

Considering the variability in iron levels in humans, this information may not benefit some.

It certainly is not necessary to go to extreme lengths to avoid all phytates in your diet. It is impossible to avoid these anti-nutrient substances totally, and that is not advised as the foods that contain them are nutritious and healthy; instead care should be taken in the method of preparation, also eating a varied diet which includes mineral rich foods, to reduce the risk of nutrient deficiency, from the action of phytic acid.

The best way of preparation to reduce the negative aspect of phytic acid or phytates and to aid the release of phosphorus that is required with calcium in the human body, is to soak beans and pulses overnight, throw away the water (there will be some mineral loss with this method) and cook thoroughly in fresh water. Another option is to add some liquid whey to help reduce mineral loss with the overnight soaking water and cook thoroughly. With wholegrains, some lemon can be added to water when cooking as porridge.

Sprouting beans and pulses can increase protein levels and help reduce the phytic acid levels, as can the process of fermentation. This is where sour dough bread with a natural starter culture, improves the mineral availability from the flour.

Lighter semi-wholegrains with a percentage of husk removed are often tolerated better by wheat-sensitive individuals. This may illustrate there being a place for semi-white wholegrains in bread and baking, providing the grain is organic and has been de-husked by cold pressed milling, that is, without the application of heat which destroys nutrients.

The whole issue of wheat is ensuring you choose a traditional variety and then experimenting whether wholegrain or semi-wholegrain best suits your digestion.

Beans contain beneficial fibre and resistant starch (not digested in the intestine) which promotes gut health and growth of healthy friendly bacteria.

Pulses and beans do not contain a full range of all eight amino acids, making these foods an incomplete protein source, but by combining pulses with wholegrains which contain complementary amino acids, they provide a source of full protein for the body's needs. With various foods eaten over the day, the body can have an ample reserve of amino acids – these foods do not need to be eaten at the same meal.

SOME HIGH PHYTATE FOODS

Sesame, linseeds, beans, almonds, brazil nuts, peanuts, soya, oats and cocoa.

Ancient tribes knew instinctively how to prepare food to reduce the negative effect of phytic acid, by soaking and fermenting their grains. Personally, I would recommend eating a variety of different grains to gain a full complement of nutrients, and to make sure the bread is naturally fermented.

THE PROBLEM WITH MODERN WHEAT

Modern wheat is indigestible and does not resemble in any way the wheat we had available decades ago. It is hybridised, cross-bred and manipulated scientifically to produce a strain of robust 'strong' wheat with a high gluten content that is good for baking purposes.

This favours the baking industry, and the UK no longer needs to rely on importing strong wheat flour from the USA or Canada.

In developing this 'super' modern wheat variety, valuable nutrients have been lost, the structure of the plant does not sway in the wind but is stockier, shorter and has a very high gluten content.

Modern wheat contains 42 chromosomes developed through programmes of cross breeding. It is the most widely grown cultivated grain throughout the world. Old fashioned traditional variety of superior nutritious wheat contained 28 chromosomes and the old wild strains only 14 chromosomes.

Modern wheat contains more of the types of gluten that can be problematic in the gut. An article in 2014 mentioned that coeliac sufferers can tolerate older wheat varieties, with a different molecular structure.[9]

It is not coincidental that the rise in gluten intolerant individuals and digestive disorders has risen in direct correlation to the world-wide consumption of modern wheat. Gluten cannot be digested and broken down easily in the human digestive tract, this can cause extreme sensitivity in some people and lead to inflammatory conditions.[10]

Certainly, this knowledge is a sign of cause and effect and needs action – if you are one of those sensitive individuals.

There are many other nutritious grains to consider, instead of the focus on wheat-based foods. Some people do well reducing or avoiding intake of grains altogether, but others may feel they have lost a rich source of complex carbohydrate (unprocessed) food which is easy to access in hectic times and that they need for energy and well-being. This requires a little experimentation on which grains suit you as an individual.

One thing is clear however; do not consume modern wheat in any form if you are suffering with digestive disorders. I would go further to say, do not consume modern wheat at all even if you feel well; it is unhealthy, causes bloating and distension in most people and has low nutritional value.

You do not have to have coeliac disease to be gluten sensitive. Research has shown that non-coeliac individuals can experience a range of symptoms and auto-immune reactions with the ingestion of wheat gluten.[11]

Systemic inflammatory processes, with compromised damaged intestinal lining, increased gut permeability and a high incidence of IBS can be found in individuals who are sensitive to wheat.

In one article, researchers concluded that less reactive species of grains were to be advised in individuals with wheat sensitivity, this can slow down development of the disease and improve quality of life.[12]

When eating rye or barley grains which contain different gliadin (gluten) strains to wheat, some people can suffer with cross reaction symptoms with inflamed bowel tissue, because the body has become sensitised through eating wheat gluten. It may take quite a while for the body to adjust. Often as time goes on, tolerance can be reached with these grains, regardless that they contain gluten. The same situation can happen when oats which do not contain gluten are grown near to wheat and have become contaminated. As sensitivity to gluten reduces, any oats may be tolerated.

In my opinion, modern wheat is generally not well tolerated, not only for its high gluten content but because repetitive cross-breeding has produced a product that human body digestive enzymes cannot recognise and if you only experience mild discomfort, such as bloating with wheat, avoid it anyway, as your body is protesting against a product that is indigestible.

A GUIDE TO CEREAL GRAINS

Ancient varieties are extremely nutritious, tasty and devoid of dubious manipulation by man. They contain natural low levels of gluten, that can be tolerated with sensitive individuals. It may be necessary, however to heal the gut, before introducing any old varieties of grain.

EMMER	This ancient grain, available today, contains beneficial levels of vitamins and minerals and protein. It can be cooked like rice and eaten with lentils or beans.
EINKORN	Another ancient grain, also rich in protein, vitamins and minerals.
KAMUT	An ancient grain, with a lovely flavour, rich in essential fatty acids and trace elements.
SPELT	An ancient grain, used by the Romans. Well tolerated by wheat sensitive people and rich in B vitamins, vitamin E, minerals and fibre.
BUCKWHEAT	Not actually a grain but a fruit flower. Highly nutritious, containing B vitamins, minerals and fibre. An excellent source of protein. Gluten-free. Makes wonderful pancakes.

MILLET	Extremely nutritious with B vitamins, vitamin A, E, rich in calcium, phosphorus and potassium. Gluten-free. Cooks like rice, or as a pudding.
QUINOA	Eaten in some parts of the world as a staple form of complete protein, (wash well, it contains saponins – a soapy substance plant chemical), rich in all the essential amino acids, potassium, iron, zinc and B vitamins. Gluten-free.
OATS	Does not contain gluten but if grown near gluten grains can become cross infected. A healthy nutrient, fibre rich food. Has a gut soothing effect.
CORN or maize	A nutritious grain, containing beta carotene, and B vitamins, calcium and trace elements. Gluten-free.
TEFF	An ancient grass grown predominately in Ethiopia. Highly nutritious, complete food. Provides many health benefits. Rich in many minerals, vitamins and protein. Gluten-free.
BARLEY	An old variety of grain, a source of protein, rich in fibre, vitamins and minerals. Contains gluten but is less reactive than wheat.
RYE	Very rich in phosphorus, potassium, minerals, especially the dark variety. Contains gluten but likely to cause less reaction than wheat.

It would be interesting and wise, to check that the source of your food is what is stated on the label; this is mindful shopping. It requires only an initial output of energy for busy city bound individuals, thereafter shopping becomes easier and the urge to grab some junk food when rushed and ravenous subsides. Hopefully you will, in your quiet moments, have stocked up on healthy snacks and goodies.

This is where the pleasure side of shopping and eating comes in. You have shopped mindfully, therefore you can relax in the knowledge that whatever item you find in your cupboards are the best the market has on offer, in pure unadulterated, unprocessed forms that had not done the rounds of the giant food processing factories.

What can be better? No more stress over what to eat, no more reaching for the quick sugar fix, the chocolate, biscuits, cake or ice-cream. No more suffering with the after effects of a sugar binge.

This is not to say goodies are to be denied. In fact, it is the opposite. Being human we all like to indulge in 'goodies', they are good for the soul, food for the mind and treats for enjoyment. The crux of the matter, however is having your goodies in a healthy form.

GOING AGAINST THE GRAIN

The 'bad' goodies can easily be converted into 'good' goodies. This is achieved with substituting the unhealthy ingredients for healthy alternatives. It may mean a little more home cooking or baking, but this is not a bad activity, even if you are not the world's greatest cook. Quick, tasty healthy snacks can be made in next to no time, even with the busiest individual. Refer to chapter 10.

Pottering in the kitchen is a marvellous stress reliever, savouring the delights of aromas and flavours can stimulate your mental awareness, awaken brain power, and is the perfect antidote to stagnating office bound activities. There is more to life than work, life should be a fine balance between productivity and relaxation.

At the centre of all this, is your digestive system. It does not thrive under stressful conditions. It is well recognised that digestive disorders generally occur more often in people with dynamic, stressful, hectic lifestyles than with calm, unstressed individuals who take time to relax when eating and have a more laid-back attitude to life.

SOUND CHOICE FOR A HEALTHY BODY

How to achieve this desired state needs time and effort to put into practice all the points that relate to your health problem. If you are unwell, it is the only answer, however to maintaining long-term health.

With determination you can get to the root cause of your health problems, you will achieve a new way at looking at food, food preparation and be able to appreciate the benefits you experience with new methods of eating, also to recognise the consequences of your old eating habits and lifestyle.

The main benefit to be gained is a calm happy digestive system. By eating in tune with − not against your digestive system − your symptoms will improve and eating once more becomes enjoyable. You will have the freedom of enjoying life to the full without constantly worrying about the effect on your digestion from the food you eat.

CHAPTER NINE

On the Road
to Digestive Health

'Not life, but good life is to be chiefly valued.'
Socrates 469 BC

REALISTIC TIMESCALE GOALS

Helping yourself to better health, is what this book is all about. The causes of digestive ill-health are the points to remember, when the spirit flags. If you make plans to deal with the basic root cause of your health problem – areas that you have identified as being applicable to your situation and are dealing with the underlying circumstances that have contributed to your current state of poor health, you can work towards the goal of reversing any damaging dietary and lifestyle factors, with confidence and determination.

Armed with knowledge – a new regard for food and a critical eye on what a healthy lifestyle offers, you can look forward to renewed health and fitness.

This reversal of damaging factors in your lifestyle, takes time. Compared to the relatively fast reaction with drug medication, nature will run at its own pace, and this varies in individuals. You may have friends who are making similar changes for their health problems and you wish to make comparison.

The rate of healing processes in the human body is completely unique, it depends on your individual biochemical body make-up. There is no magic formula that gets you from being sick, to a fit person, within a given timescale. You should however be making progress day by day and feeling better within a few weeks after making the necessary dietary changes.

REGRESSION WHILST PROGRESSING

It is best to work with your body, listening and watching for signs of progress or regression. When negative signs appear after a period of healing progress, this is perfectly normal. It is an indication, that the body needs time to catch up with itself.

As the body heals, digests and absorbs food in an improved state, gently detoxifies, utilises nutrients at the cellular level, the liver needs to be acting in tandem with this progress. As the liver is the largest main organ of metabolic activity, it may get slightly overwhelmed in its vital functions, depending on what doses and form of supplementation is used in the healing programme.

This is a time for you to step back, enjoy the break and give time for the body to adjust. This is best taken over a day or two, when all supplementation should be stopped, dietary changes should stay in place, and plenty of water taken to help the body cleanse. When feeling back in form, re-start the supplements, first at the lowest dose, then increasing back to the recommended dose.

There are occasions where sudden discontinuation of damaging foods or drink can cause a rebound effect. The body has 'coped' dealing with undesirable dietary items, perhaps for a long while, and suddenly it does not have this challenge. In my experience, this positive regulated *all out-way forward* is the best, regardless of a few days of withdrawal symptoms. 'Prolonging the agony' in a long drawn out process, of reducing instead of avoiding problem food and drinks, can result in reduced healing time, and a loss of peace of mind. The will to succeed is delayed and ultimately may be lost, which defeats the issue. Changes to diet and lifestyle should be dealt with positively, without trying to delay the outcome.

COMPLIANCE WITH PROFESSIONAL RECOMMENDATIONS

Compliance with practitioner recommendations is part of your insurance of success with any programme you may be on. I have experienced some cases where, delighted with improved digestion, some people feel that – a little of this and a little of that – with some forbidden food, will not upset the strict regime they are on.

This is the wrong move to make, the digestive system is very finely tuned, only when it is fully healed and robust, is there the possibility of tolerating the occasional unhealthy food. These actions can set the programme back, as after all, allowing challenging, gut irritating food or drink into an area of the body, that is trying to heal, is counter-productive.

POTENTIAL PROBLEMS IN ADJUSTING TO NEW IDEALS

It is well recognised that peer pressure plays a part in your ability to follow the strict regime necessary, to reverse and heal your digestive health symptoms.

There is only one answer to this sometimes, upsetting situation. Critical individuals do not have to live with your constant health problems. Nor do they have to experience your daily struggle with health and the constant worry over what to eat and the stress of dealing with how your gut may react to certain allergenic foods. Friends should respect your wishes and have patience to understand your views.

Caring individuals will understand, family and work colleagues should understand, at the end of the day, you have one body, one life and you need to learn how to live in a fashion that does not challenge your body, allowing it to have the chance to heal and reverse symptoms of ill health. If this means avoiding popular foods in a social setting, it should not mean loss of face or friendship as a result, if it does then question that friendship.

You are the one to gain and you have nothing to lose. Ignoring stressful individuals can calm the mind and reduce stress on your digestive system. It is simply not worth throwing away the promise of improved health, for the chance of a binge now and then as there will always be a price to pay.

Accepting new lifestyle ideas is a challenging thought, but also enlightening and exciting. The belief in getting well again, is a reward to set your sights on.

IT IS NOT SUCH A BIG ISSUE WITH A NEW REGIME

Should doubts or questions in your mind be bothering you then discuss them with your practitioner, or if you are working on self-help recommendations in this book, re-read sections that may supply the answers.

There are many other excellent books on digestive health, with the functional, and nutritional medicine approach, that can offer further support in confirmation of facts.

Keep calm, focused and enjoy your body's journey to better health, in the knowledge that you have taken your health into your hands and are in control of the outcome.

In the work environment, take in a healthy lunchbox, with supportive healthy snacks for the times when you become so hungry from your work load and energy output that you may run the risk of slipping into the old bad dietary habits.

TROUBLESHOOTING BASICS

If enjoying eating out with friends and colleagues, do not despair that you cannot or will not be able to eat foods that you know are unhealthy. There are always relatively healthy choices of food available: gluten-free pizza for instance, omelettes, soups, salads with healthy protein. It may not be organic, but that will not matter, you can eat organic at home, the focus is that the right type of foods can be eaten without posing a threat to your digestive system.

Arm yourself with a mental list of allowable foods, and a word to chefs, who can prove quite willing to offer you some food items of your choice. Most chefs are aware of the rising incidence of digestive health problems and most restaurants are very willing to support you. Do not shy away from asking. It is an acceptable request these days.

If you do fall by the wayside by chance, do not despair, the body is very forgiving and will re-start the process of healing. The only drawback however, is that, repeatedly falling into former habits shows a lack of commitment, and from a time point of view, it could put back your healing programme by weeks or months.

We are, in fact, armed with a whole array of body hormones that our body uses to fight disease and control symptoms of sickness. It just requires us supplying the right food to support the actions of this amazing system. Nature provides just about everything required to keep us healthy, providing we do not challenge the system too often with man-made options. Modern day living offers many damaging temptations that can be hard to resist, but everyone must make their own choices and pay with whatever consequences come their way.

THE NATURAL HEALING FORCE WITHIN

Do not lose touch with the ability of your body to heal and the amazing properties in the food you eat. It is generally thought we need to eat to survive and that food supplies sufficient calories to fill the stomach and give us energy to fulfil that role – there is much more to eating than that.

Few people would imagine that your mind and body require food to nourish all body cells, as building blocks for new cells and to heal symptoms of ill health. The healing chemicals contained in food or botanical plants also provide you with an alternative natural pharmacy source to pharmaceutical drug treatment.

NATURAL HEALING PROPERTIES IN FOODS AND HERBS:

- Antimicrobials
- Anti-inflammatories
- Antioxidants
- Antiseptic agents
- Antibiotics
- Demulcents (rich in mucilage that soothes irritated tissues)
- Hormone regulators
- Detoxifiers
- Anti-stressors
- Anti-ageing agents
- Digestive stimulants
- Sedatives
- Nerve tonics
- Choleretics (improving bile flow)
- Blood purifiers
- Immune regulators

I stress that we are talking here about minor health problems and chronic poor health not acute or emergency medical cases that require a doctor's skill and medication.

Foods contain remarkable healing powers over and above the nutrients and calories provided in your daily diet. The body uses this food with the combined effort of the brain, the gut and all the thousand chemical reactions in the body.

THE POWER OF THE MIND:
THE PLACEBO, NOCEBO EFFECT

The considerable significance of the mind helping to heal the body cannot be emphasised enough. Emotional stress can cause hormonal havoc in a body undergoing healing processes.

Keeping in the right frame of mind, with the belief that you can conquer your poor state of health, will help you tap into your own body pharmacy. The subconscious mind helps the body release opiates, neurotransmitters and other chemicals, in response to pain, inflammation and discomfort.

These processes work by the power of thought processes in the brain affecting the physical metabolism in the body. The brain and the gut are intrinsically biochemically linked. If you believe you will get better, your digestion has a better chance of improving.

These expectations are linked to what is known as the placebo effect, widely used in drug trials. A belief in the power of the mind over the body, a belief so powerful that it can influence the release of a cascade of chemicals which then address symptoms of poor health.

This effect was described in an article by Erik Vance in the *National Geographic* magazine 2016, demonstrating medical trials for research on neurochemical mechanisms. Patients given a placebo (dummy pill) had been found to show improvement in health, that matched patients on drug therapy, and furthermore that placebos work also when the patient is aware they are not on the real treatment.[1]

Vance also mentions a 2010 research trial at Harvard Medical School, after 21 days of taking a placebo, people with IBS were reported as feeling remarkably better when compared with people who had received no treatment at all.

In contrast, the nocebo effect is when expectations are so low within a person's mind that the opposite outcome can be the result and symptoms get worse.

As this demonstrates, it would not be wise to let peer pressure distract you from your single-minded approach in following a programme to improve your diet and change a damaging lifestyle.

As many medical tests on the placebo effect demonstrate, information taken from environment and social relationships can have a profound influence on emotions and health-related outcomes in healing processes. If surrounded by supportive individuals, your mind can be conditioned to expect a positive outcome in your journey to cure and heal your digestive disorder.

KEEP POSITIVE AND BELIEVE IN YOURSELF

With the correct mind-set, if you can tap into this aspect of healing, you can be assured of an increased chance of a successful result in any treatment plan. It is proven science – the brain directs the healing. One has only to consider the effect of body contact and animal therapy with the elderly and in hospitals: a positive, contented, happy mind can help the healing process, reduce inflammation and pain and help to cure disease.

Research is constantly revealing, not only links between the nutritional value of food in relation to health, but the hundreds of new plant chemicals that influence metabolism, discovered in various kinds of food. These have been found to offer extraordinary health benefits from reducing cholesterol, fighting heart disease and degenerative disorders to healing the gut. You can apply this knowledge, in your own personal situation, healing with food and plants and using diet to achieve a reversal of symptoms of chronic poor health, in a manner which does not harm the body but nourishes it.

YOUR HEALTH IN YOUR HANDS

Quite simply, what we eat affects quality of health, the correct diet for your body is your passport to good health. Not only do we have healing chemicals within the body, but a whole arsenal from nature's store. Used with the appropriate professional advice, these pharmacological properties in food and herbs, can be utilised to provide all the natural treatment the body requires.

Choosing the wrong diet can cause you to miss months if not years of active healthy life. Getting well again requires all factors pertaining to health, being addressed. A chronic state of poor health can take years to develop, and without action taken to reverse the situation, matters can only get worse.

As you can see, there is a lot to consider and plenty of areas in your life that may require improvement. Your health is really in your hands. With changes put in place, you can achieve a new level of well-being, and huge self-satisfaction in having followed your instincts and cleared up your own health problems: an achievement to be proud of.

LOOK TO THE FUTURE – KEEP ON COURSE

It is a misconception that health, once gained can continue to be maintained with little effort. If you return to unhealthy habits, it is likely your body will repeat the chain of events that caused you to become unwell in the first place, if you falter in your reserve to make dietary and lifestyle changes a permanent feature in your life, then you are failing to recognise your body's needs and are more than likely looking for a quick fix without planning for the changes to be long-term.

Hopefully with the help of this book, you will appreciate what actions are necessary to clear up your digestive health disorders. You may still have a long way to go, until you feel you are digesting well and do not suffer food sensitivity or other distressing gastrointestinal problems.

Do not ponder on the time ahead of you, rather concentrate on the present and how far you have travelled from the past, in terms of improvement in health.

If you have seen encouraging results, however small – you are on the correct path.

By giving in to temptation, consider if you can risk undoing all the benefit you have achieved. If you have successfully applied the recommendations in this book? It is not worth throwing away the experience gained.

For long-term maintenance of good health, you need to continue, not just with a new diet but a new way of looking at how to keep healthy. To be environmentally aware of the dangers of chemicals in diet, body-care products, water and, of many other factors posing a risk to health, including electro-magnetic fields (EMFs). Our polluted world and increasing use of damaging technology, can give rise to stress, but try to reduce the overall load your body is exposed to.

A person who is unwell cannot enjoy life fully or the companionship of friends in a social setting. Some people feel obliged, or are forced by peer pressure, to participate socially, and return to old habits, despite feeling ill by doing so. As the old diet and lifestyle factors have been found to be the root cause of your digestive health problems, some thought needs to be given to a situation that is having a negative effect on your health.

CHAPTER TEN

Dietary Summary and
Recipe Ideas for Optimum Health

'Each of the substances of a man's diet,
acts upon his body and changes it in some way,
and upon these changes his whole life depends.'
Hippocrates 460 BC

IDEAL DAILY FOOD BALANCE ON THE AVERAGE PLATE

Allowances should be made for individually tailored dietary plans.

55% should be carbohydrates as **wholegrains, pulses, legumes, fruit, vegetables and salad**, with half of your plate containing vegetables and salad. Fresh fruit salad should be eaten daily.

30% should be fats made up of 10% saturated animal fat and 20% essential polyunsaturated and monounsaturated fats as **nuts, seeds, oily fish and unprocessed vegetable oils**.

15% should be protein as **fish, meat, eggs, dairy, grain and pulse combinations**.

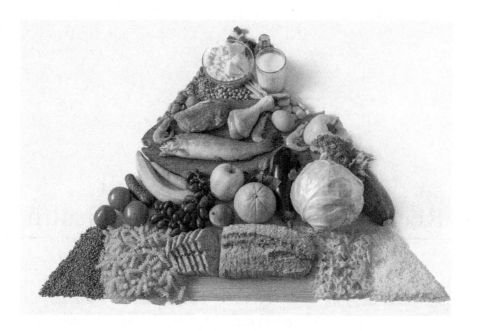

EAT ORGANIC, WHOLEFOOD, SUGAR FREE, UNPROCESSED AND ADDITIVE-FREE PRODUCE

WATER

Our body is at least 60% water. Water is the medium for all body processes, it lubricates every cell. It is required for the heart to beat efficiently, for healthy circulation and is involved in digestion, absorption and elimination. It is the most important part of any treatment therapy; you can live longer without food than water, it is the essential factor for life itself. Without it, no body system can work and if it is in short supply, you can experience headaches, muscle aches and pains, dizziness, lack of concentration and loss of coordination. It is a critical requirement in the elderly, who, with the ageing process, lose elasticity in the skin and the ability to hydrate properly.

Hydrate regularly throughout the day. It doesn't take much to become dehydrated. As soon as you feel thirsty, it is already a good hour after you have become dehydrated. Water is continuously lost in the process of breathing, this can represent about a half pint of fluid loss, so it must be regularly replaced.

HEALTHY FOOD PREPARATION TIPS:

Do not peel organic potatoes, carrots, apples and other produce, just scrub clean. There are nutrients within the skin and plenty of healthy fibre.

Steam vegetables in a little water with a lid on to preserve vitamins which can evaporate in steam. Keep cooking water to use in sauces, not to throw down the sink, it contains healthy amounts of potassium and nutrients that the body needs.

Never barbecue food until it is overly brown or burnt. This produces acrylamide, a carcinogenic substance that is damaging to cells. The same thing happens in browning of chips, crisps and toasting bread. You can have healthy oven chips, home-made, sprinkled with avocado oil.

Avoid cutting fruit or vegetables long before eating or cooking. Oxidation (the browning and spoiling of food that takes place) will cause nutrient loss.

Avoid prolonged high heat cooking; nutrients are destroyed. Particularly the white protein content of eggs, and the structure of meat. All heat from cooking destroys vital enzymes in fresh produce, so blanch or keep the produce al dente, with a bite to it, and cook for as short a time as possible. Soggy overcooked food, lacking all its original colour is pretty much lifeless and lacking in nutrients.

Healthy cooking does not take time, compared to the time it takes to follow instructions to a special recipe. Obviously on special occasions, it is lovely to indulge in special dishes, but for everyday cooking, the main necessity is learning how to combine healthy combinations of colourful food and cooking it simply and with the least attention to time. Lightly cooked foods are healthy, (pork and chicken must be well-cooked though), certainly vegetables lightly semi-steamed for a few minutes are nutrient rich and delicious.

With the abundant TV chef programmes, you may feel duty bound to produce a masterpiece with everyday main meals. This is not necessary, if you look carefully, the mass of sugar, salt and unhealthy items flung into pots, the high cooking temperatures and the loss of nutrients in cooking methods, do not make for a healthy meal. There are exceptions of course, this is a generalised observation.

The best meals are simply prepared, with attention to detail for nutritional content, colour and flavour. Home-made quick sauces with crème fraiche or yoghurt, green herbs and red and green pesto can add to the end effect.

Wholefoods are more satisfying, they take longer to digest, help balance blood sugar levels, supply energy and are naturally high in nutrients, making them tastier (the flavour is in the nutrients). When additives and artificial flavourings are added to highly processed food, it is because man has destroyed the nutrients in the manufacturing processes and they need synthetically replacing.

In supermarkets – keep a beady eye on positioning of organic goods on the shelves. Oils will spoil when placed close to overhead heating or with exposure to bright light, they are best also in a dark container.

Un-packaged or non vacuum-packed foods are less likely to be contaminated from plastic packaging. Unblended honey from bees which are not sugar fed in winter (heat treatment for blending can reduce nutrient content) – is the sort of food that you should be looking for. Having the organic label is not enough, you need to delve deeper as to the production methods.

Digestive disorders do not just appear out of the blue, they develop as a direct result of poor diet and hectic lifestyle. Some people are obviously more genetically prone than others and are at a disadvantage here, but once well again, finding the balance that suits you as an individual, will serve to keep you in good health.

SUGGESTIONS FOR A HEALTHY BREAKFAST:

BIRCHERMUESLI: Adapted from a recipe formulated by Dr Maximilian Bircher-Benner (1867–1939) in a clinic in the Swiss Alps, who originally used apples, nuts, dried fruit and oats and advocated a high intake of raw food.

Fresh organic fruit salad with a colourful range of fruits; blueberries, raspberries, apples, pears, citrus fruit, bananas and any fruit in season, with sun ripened mangoes and papaya.

Nuts and seeds – almonds, walnuts, hazelnuts, brazils, cashews and seeds, sunflower, pumpkin, hempseeds, linseeds, coconut, dates, figs.

Sugar-free plain live yoghurt plus sugar-free, wheat-free muesli. Quark can also be used in place of yoghurt.

Chop and mix all the above together in a bowl, add a measure of 100% organic pure fruit juice, the mixture should be creamy. Pomegranate juice would give added nutritional value.

This makes a refreshing good start to the day, takes hours to fully digest, contains complex carbohydrates, fats and protein, to help blood sugar balance and provides numerous flavonoids and plant chemicals for the day ahead. It is a recipe that encourages glucose storage for maintaining energy throughout the day.

The feedback I usually hear with this suggested breakfast choice, is that a morning snack is unnecessary because the substantial nutritious breakfast sees people through until lunchtime. Eating protein at each meal helps balance blood sugar levels and helps to stop cravings.

Millet and oat porridge, made with rice, or nut milk, served with ground almonds, coconut, berries, and crème fraiche or quark is another option for cold days.

Amounts are deliberately not given, judge portions for the number of persons eating.

SUPER FUNCTIONAL FOODS TO BOOST ENERGY, COMBAT STRESS AND AID DETOXIFICATION

FOR A FORTIFIED NUTRITIOUS START TO THE DAY

ADD TO BIRCHERMUESLI:

A green powder mix of organic split cell chlorella and spirulina, containing a form of protein, vitamins, minerals and essential fatty acids, with more calcium than milk, higher B12 levels than other food, iron and a rich source of chlorophyll and magnesium. This powder is best mixed with yoghurt as microalgae can enhance the beneficial effect of a fermented milk product by increasing the level of acid-forming bacteria. Health benefits have been well documented, showing increased immune and liver detoxification support, stress reduction, anti-tumour and anti-viral activity. Caution in pregnancy – detoxification is not advisable.

Organic pre-sprouted barley grass powder. A nutritious source of protein, vitamins, minerals and trace elements.

Hemp powder. Contains high levels of complete protein and essential fatty acids, fibre and iron. Make certain you source a quality-controlled superior unprocessed product.

Indian gooseberry powder known as amla, a rich source of vitamin C and **acai Brazilian berry.** Vitamin C supports the immune system by helping the action of white blood cells to fight foreign invaders.

Bee pollen granules. These contain practically all known nutrients required by humans. It is extremely high in protein, contains nectar and enzymes, flavonoids and is a true super food noted in many studies to provide benefit for numerous health problems. Caution in pregnancy.

Bee propolis powder. Always source additive-free, organic bee products. This product is the bee 'glue' that is used as a sealer in bee hive structure. It contains essential oils, resin, protein, vitamins, minerals and flavonoids and is well recognised as having anti-microbial properties. Caution in pregnancy.

Organic kelp powder rich in calcium, magnesium, iodine and trace elements. Caution and professional advice required if suffering with hyperthyroid, hypertension or cardiovascular health problems.

Optional:

A dash of lemon juice to aid absorption of iron and calcium.

Grated ginger root to aid digestion and act as an anti-inflammatory agent.

Cinnamon powder to support blood sugar balance.

This breakfast is best made up in a family-size bowl, amounts and choice of ingredients added can vary according to taste, it should be a creamy mixture neither too sour or too bland.

Experiment each day with different fruits of compatible flavours, a variety of pure juices with nutritional value. As the juice is mixed with complex carbohydrates in wholegrains, the instant quick 'sugar effect' is minimised. Creamy mixtures from dairy or coconut cream can create diversity in your daily super mix.

For sceptics, a week on proper home-made Bichermuesli and not just from a cardboard box, may be convincing enough in terms of increased energy, concentration and feeling of well-being.

In answer to the many comments I noted from people who are focused on 'fast food' options and insist it may be too time consuming to prepare, I can assure readers once you have all ingredients available, it is just a matter of filling a bowl and stirring!

The amount of nutrients supplied for your daily energy needs, contained in this type of breakfast, cannot in any way be compared to a slice of toast or a bowl of ready-made muesli from a cardboard packet. This approach to eating will revitalise your gut environment and improve digestive function. Having convinced people to try this breakfast option, I have yet to see anyone who didn't feel revitalised.

HEALTHY WEEKEND OPTIONS:

Buckwheat, chestnut and almond flour pancakes, made with egg and served with fresh berries and yoghurt or crème fraiche.

Scrambled, poached or boiled eggs with wheat-free wholemeal toast, with healthy smoothies based on fresh fruit, nut milk, juice plus the super functional food powders.

Grilled tomatoes, mushrooms, organic healthy sausage, with herb omelette and healthy smoothie as above.

LUNCH SUGGESTIONS:

- Eating a raw enzyme-rich mixed salad daily can help increase digestibility of foods
- Colourful mixed salad; avocado, dark and light green lettuce, watercress, celery, coloured mixed peppers, cucumber, tomatoes, taken with a portion of protein; fish, egg, pulses, meat or dairy
- Additive-free organic lentil, fish, meat or vegetable soup, wheat-free wholemeal bread plus a portion of protein; cheese or egg
- Baked potatoes with olive oil, a protein filling; cottage cheese and beans, cheese and pineapple
- Gluten-free pizza with sardines, anchovies, seafood or meat in the topping
- Mushrooms, fish or eggs on wheat-free toast
- Omelettes with vegetables and protein

DINNER SUGGESTIONS:

Each meal to contain carbohydrate, fat and protein.

- Wild and wholegrain rice risotto with steamed mixed vegetables, olive oil, garlic, onions, prawns, seafood and parmesan cheese
- Stuffed dark green cabbage leaves with minced beef, lemon

juice, cumin, olives, pine nuts, garlic and onions, served with quinoa or wholegrain rice

- Chicken ragout in mushroom and quark sauce, served with broccoli, mashed potatoes and carrots
- Sliced potatoes, nutmeg, garlic, olive oil and yoghurt in alternate layers – baked in oven, served with steamed salmon in lemon juice and watercress or peas
- Wheat-free pasta with minced meat, seafood or fish in tomato, cheese or yoghurt and basil sauce with garlic, onions, herbs, olive oil
- Mousakka made with alternatively sliced aubergines, potatoes, tomatoes, minced meat, herbs, olive oil, garlic and cheese sauce, baked in the oven and served with greens

HEALTHY DESERT SUGGESTIONS:

- Pureed whips; avocado, mango, bananas, berries, pears with crème fraiche, quark or cream
- Baked bananas with almonds, cinnamon and whipped cream
- Rhubarb or apple fruit crumble with gluten or wheat-free topping made with grains, ground nuts, coconut butter or butter and coconut sugar, served with cream
- Baked filled apples with sultanas, honey and walnuts served with yoghurt
- Chestnut and buckwheat pancakes with fresh fruit and cream
- Apple rings and cinnamon dipped in wheat-free batter and fried gently in butter or coconut fat, served with home-made sugar-free ice-cream

NUTRITIOUS GLUTEN-FREE FLOUR VARIETIES

Chestnut flour, almond flour, coconut flour, buckwheat flour, quinoa flour, amaranth flour, chickpea flour, corn flour, hempseed flour, rice flour, lentil flour, flaxseed flour, potato flour, pea flour.

Any combinations of flour can give positive results; I offer only recipe ideas, not recipes, using different ingredient choices to encourage experimentation.

This method of cooking and baking can increase the nutrient value of your meal, simply by not repeatedly eating the same foods in a favourite recipe and recognising the many different foods available, that you may never have tried.

It may be a question of experimentation with different ingredients, but you can gain benefit by designing a recipe that suits your digestion and personal tastes. If it turns out not so perfect a result, at least you know the ingredients are the healthiest and can be adapted next time. Weights and measures are not given. Required amounts for a meal are so variable. This is not a recipe book but is designed to give information as to the nutritional content of food and how to incorporate these nutrient rich foods into your diet.

GLUTEN WHEAT YEAST - FREE BREAD:

POPPADOMS: chickpea flour, lentil flour, bicarbonate of soda, add a touch of apple cider vinegar to activate the bicarbonate, cumin, sea-salt, pepper, hempseed oil.

Work together with water into a dough, to produce flatbread, gentle fry or cook on a griddle.

FOCCACIA: rice flour, corn flour, almond flour, bicarbonate of soda, a touch of apple cider vinegar, sunflower seeds, a little rice milk, olive oil, cumin, garlic powder, black pepper, chunky sea-salt, olives.

Kneed all ingredients together, adjusting for consistency – not too sticky or too dry, adding more, or less, flour and liquid. Flatten, prick with fork, sprinkle with sea-salt and chopped olives, drizzle with olive oil, bake in oven.

BUCKWHEAT AND FLAXSEED ROLLS: buckwheat flour, flaxseed flour, potato flour, sea-salt, pepper, bicarbonate of soda, a little flax oil, 1 spoon yoghurt or apple cider vinegar.

Kneed and form with water into rolls, sprinkle with linseeds and bake.

CORNBREAD: almond flour, golden maize or corn flour, sea-salt, bicarbonate of soda, apple cider vinegar, poppy seeds, a beaten egg.

Mix all ingredients with water to an oval shape, sprinkle with poppy seeds and bake.

AMARANTH, CHESTNUT AND POTATO BREAD: amaranth flour, chestnut flour, potato flour, sea-salt and pepper, bicarbonate of soda, apple cider vinegar, onion powder, mixed herbs.

Mix with water, sprinkle with pumpkin seeds and bake in loaf tin.

RAISIN, ALMOND SODA BREAD: almond flour, raisins, sea-salt, bicarbonate of soda, eggs, a little honey, apple cider vinegar, buttermilk.

Mix to a round shape, make 2 large cross cuts on top, brush with buttermilk, sprinkle with gluten-free oats and bake.

If tolerated, the above grain recipe ideas can be used with yeast and honey to activate, instead of baking soda and apple cider vinegar as a raising agent.

There are many combinations you can use with the above grains and herbs, sweet spices, nuts and seeds to experiment with. Wholegrain unprocessed flours need more fluid and some form of oil and fat from dairy, to improve palatability and to produce a good consistency for cutting. Buttermilk is good for these properties as well as providing flavour.

SOURDOUGH BREAD IDEAS:

Fermentation helps to make grains digestible, it helps to break down the phytic acid and release the calcium. It is possible to buy starter cultures from artisan bakeries or you can make your own by mixing a half cup of flour, rye, spelt or rice with a little warm water, mix to a paste and leave to ferment for 12–24 hours. When it bubbles, the fermentation process has begun. Fermented sourdough bread made with gluten-free grains, is extremely nourishing and improves health of the gut microbiome. Lactic acid bacteria – liquid whey can also be used for bread making. Sour cream, buttermilk or yoghurt can be added to the bread mixture with bicarbonate of soda in place of a culture.

HEALTHY GRAIN OPTIONS OR COMBINATIONS FOR SOURDOUGH BREAD:

Rye, barley, spelt, buckwheat, einkorn, kamut, teff, emmer with a percentage added of gram or chickpea flour, potato, rice, corn or pea flour, if desired. Experiment with various combinations, try to combine lighter flours with heavier varieties and enrich with oils, buttermilk or butter; sourdough bread is more nutritious and beneficial for improving digestion and maintaining a healthy gut.

QUICK AND EASY CAKES:

Melt half a block of butter in a saucepan, cool, add 2 tablespoons of honey or coconut sugar. Whisk 2 eggs, add to cooled mixture, 1 packet of baking powder, approximately 6 heaped large tablespoons of flour, 2 tablespoons of ground almonds, half a cup of apple juice. Mix well, this is your basic cake mixture, always adjust flour and liquid, the mixture should be creamy, light and easy to spoon into baking tin.

For flavourings: vary, either two mashed bananas plus cinnamon powder, raisins plus mixed spice, chopped mandarins with peel plus almond slivers, grated lemon rind with juice and poppy seeds, blueberries, chopped dates and walnuts plus molasses and mixed spice, chopped apples plus cloves, pineapple pieces with coconut, candied ginger chopped soaked and drained to eliminate the sugar plus ginger spice, ground hazelnuts and raspberries, pureed rhubarb, carob powder, chopped pears plus aniseed spice, chopped mangoes plus coconut, grated carrots and lemon juice.

Gluten-free flour suitable for cakes: almond flour, coconut flour (used in moderation), spelt flour, chestnut flour, rice and potato flour. Any combination depending on the result you are seeking, they are best mixed and matched, because of the different properties in each grain. A lighter sponge type of cake would be achieved with almond and spelt flour or chestnut and potato flour. Coconut flour requires a lot more fluid and should be used in combination as one cup to the main flour used.

QUICK AND EASY BISCUITS:

Melt half a pack of butter in a sauce pan, cool. Add 2 tablespoons of coconut sugar and 6 tablespoons of mixed flour chosen from the above list. The mixture should be quite stiff, add one beaten egg and flavourings – lemon drops, currants, vanilla, coconut, spices or just leave plain. Form flat small circles on tin and bake in medium oven. Ginger and blackstrap molasses as flavourings are quite delicious.

QUICK AND EASY TREATS:

Popsicles for summer. Mash avocados and mangoes separately, mix with whipped cream, crème fraiche or yoghurt, a little honey and pour alternate layers in lollipop forms and freeze. Or make ice-cream, using pistachio nuts, mashed avocado, bananas, honey, cream or crème fraiche, freeze and whip once during process.

Pancakes or pikelets made with chestnut flour and spelt or almond flour and buckwheat, with bicarbonate and a dash of lemon, to make them fluffy. Cook in butter and serve with a dribble of maple syrup or honey.

SNACKS:

Flapjacks – Melt butter, add chopped dates, blackstrap molasses, lemon juice, soften on low heat, when cooled add 2 eggs to bind, desiccated coconut and oats to form a firm sticky mixture. Press into flat tin, bake, cut into squares. Coconut pyramids – mix coconut, carob flour, ground almonds, egg white, and coconut sugar, bake until lightly brown. Softened figs in orange juice, mixed with ground almonds, and coconut flour, egg yolk and grated orange rind, coat in carob powder and bake in tin with small truffle forms.

There are many options and interesting ways of making your diet enjoyable and much more adventurous than it probably was. Experimenting with quick recipe ideas broadens your scope to enjoy your meals without being tied down to hours in the kitchen, unless of course you are a budding chef who loves that life.

SUMMARY:

The purpose of this book has been to offer support for individuals suffering from chronic digestive disorders. It does not replace medical advice but offers readers solutions to their problems that they may be unaware of. My advice should be used in conjunction with medical diagnosis where appropriate.

There are obviously many types of symptoms involved in digestive disorders and the intention of my recommendations is to help point you in the right direction to get your problems sorted, and to demonstrate the successes I have witnessed over the years in my clinics.

If comprehensive supplementation is planned as self-help, (other than just the basic support), either with herbal medicine or with nutritional products that may be sourced over the internet, professional help should be obtained, to verify quality and purity of the products and to help guide you through the many changes that could occur as the body phases through healing processes. This can be a confusing stressful complex area for an individual but a perfectly normal expected response to an experienced practitioner.

Having explained the basic physiology and biochemistry involved in digestive function, the latter part of the book is designed to give you many options for eating healthily once your health problems have cleared and you feel able to put back in foods that you previously may have had difficulty with.

The message I am hoping to convey, is that eating can be enjoyable without fast junk food. There is even more choice out there than the unhealthy mono-diets some people typically eat. Your state of health is related exactly to what food choices you put in your body.

I sincerely wish that you – the reader, gain – hope – inspiration and ultimately a full recovery.

For any further individual contact advice, please refer to my website: https://www.gjgbionutrition.org.

References

CHAPTER ONE

1. Duckett, J. (2016) 'Gastrointestinal Remedies Industry Report'. *Mintel Press Office.* (online).

2. Harding, M. (2014) 'Irritable Bowel Syndrome'. *Patient.info* (online).

3. Kaplan, G. (2015) 'The Global Burden of IBD: from 2015-2025 '. *Nature Reviews Gastroenterology & Hepatology.* (online)¬: 720-727. doi:10.1038/nr gastro.2015.150.

4. Lim, E. et al., (2015) 'Early Dynamics of the Human Gut Virome and Bacterial Microbiome in Infants'. *Natural Medicine,* 2015 Oct 21(10): 1228-34. doi:10.1038/nm.3950.

5. Clemente, J. et al., (2012) 'The Impact of the Gut Microbiota on Human Health: an integrative view'. *Cell,* Vol 148, Issue 6: 1258-1270.

6. Devkota, S. (2016) 'Gut Microbiota Research and Practice'. *Science,* Vol 35, Issue 6272: 452-453. doi:10.1126/Science.

7. Guinane, C. and Carter, P. (2013) 'Role of the Gut microbiota in health and chronic gastrointestinal disease: understanding a hidden metabolic organ'. *Therapy Advanced Gastroenterology.* 2013 Jul; 6(4): 295-380.

CHAPTER TWO

1. Jones, R. (2010) 'GP's have no difficulty dealing with symptoms of major digestive disorders, however they feel less confident when dealing with minor chronic digestive ill-health'. *Med Econnect and YOUGOV* (online) CORE UK report.

2. 'What chemicals are in cigarette smoke?' (2015) *Medical News* today/com/articles/215420.php. July 2015.

3. Bebbington, T, (2013) 'Modern day Brits becoming hunter grabbers'. *Web M.D.UK* Health News Survey for GUT week.

4. Hamzelou, J. (2013) 'Secrets of the Body'. *New Scientist*; article. Vol 217, Issue 2908: 35 -48.

5. 'Chemical Exposure in our daily lives' (2015) *Nut Sci* article and video documentary. *Mercola.com* (online).

6. Muncke, J. Peterson Meyers, J. Scheringer, M. Porta, M. (2014) 'Food packaging and migration of food contact materials: will epidemiologists rise to the neotoxic challenge?' *Journal of Epidemiology and Community Health*, 2014 (in press). doi:10.1136/jech -2013-202593.

7. Pizzorno, J. Jn. (2015) 'The Personalisation of care achievable through Patients with Gastroesophageal Reflux Disease and their Effect on Quality of Life'. World Journal of Gastroenterology. 2015 April 14: 21(14): 4302-4309. doi:10.3748/wig.v.21i114.4302.

CHAPTER THREE

1. Heidelbaugh, J. Kin, A. et al., (2012) 'Overutilization of proton-pump inhibitors: What the Clinicians need to know'. *Journal of Gastroenterology*. Jul; 4 (4): 219-232. doi:10.1177/1756283x12437358.

2. UHN Staff. (2017) 'Low Stomach Acid: A Surprising Cause of Indigestion Symptoms'. *University Health News* Mar 14, 2017. Canada.

3. English, J. (2013) 'Gastric balance: heartburn not always caused by excess acid'. *Nutrition Review* article (online) April 222013.

4. Banoo, H. Nusrat, N. et al., (2016). 'Implications of low Stomach Acid: An Update'. RAMA University. *Journal of Medical Science.* 2016;2(2):16-26.

5. Song, E. Jung, H. and Jung, J. (2013) 'The Association Between Reflux Esophagitis and Psychosocial Stress' *Journal of Digestive Diseases and Sciences.* 2013 Feb;58(20: 471-477. (online) 2012 Sept 22. doi:10. 1007/s10620-012-2377-2.

6. Yang, X-J. Jiang, H. et al., (2015) 'Anxiety and Depression in Patients with Gastroesophageal Reflux Disease and their Effect on Quality of Life'. *World Journal of Gastroenterology.* 2015 April; 21(14): 4302-4309. doi:10.3748/wjg. V21.114.4302.

CHAPTER FOUR

1. Jones, D. Hoffman, L. Quinn, S. (2011) 'Twenty First Century Medicine: A New Model for Medical Education and Practice' 137page white paper pub. *The Institute for Functional Medicine.* Spring 2009.

2. Pizzorno, J. (2012) 'Clinical Decision Making – A Functional Medicine Perspective'. *Journal Global Advances in Health and Medicine.* 2012 Sept 1 (4): 8-13. (online) doi:10.7453/gahmij.2012.1.1.002.

3. Null, G. Dean, C. et al., (2015) 'Death by Medicine'. *The Journal of Orthomolecular Medicine.* Vol 20, No 1, 2005. (online) video upload Oct 23. 2015.

4. Rohsmann, P. (2006) 'MT: A Highly Individual, Fine-Tuned Nutritional Guideline'. *Positive Health Online, Integrative Medicine for the 21st Century.* Oct 2006.

5. Kristal, H. (2002) 'The Nutrition Solution - A Guide to your Metabolic Type'. *North Atlantic Books.*

6. De Winter, B. Van den Wijngaard, R. de Jonge, W. (2012) 'Intestinal Mast Cells in Gut Inflammation and Motility Disturbance' *Science Direct*. Vol 1822, Issue1. Jan.2012. 66-73.

7. Mainz, L. Novak, N. (2007) 'Histamine and Histamine Intolerance'. Article. *American Society for Clinical Nutrition*.

8. Dave, N. Xiang, L. et al., ((2010) 'Stress and Allergic Diseases'. *Immunology Allergy Clinical North Am*. National Library of Medicine. doi:10. 1016/j.jac,2010.09.009.

9. Itan, Y. (2010) 'A Worldwide Correlation of Lactase Persistence Phenotype and Geno types' Feb 6, 2010. BMC *'Evolutionary Biology'*

10. Baron, S. (1996) 'Medical Microbiology'. Fourth edition. *Addison Wesley Publishing Company Inc*. 1996.

11. Rashidul, H. (2007) 'Human Intestinal Parasites' Dec; 25(4): 387-391 *Journal of Health, Population and Nutrition*

12. Ziffer, L. Highet, R. Klayman, D. (2015) 'Artemisinine an Endoperoxidic Antimalarial from Artemisia Annua'. 1997; Vol 72: 121-214. Progress in the Chemistry of Organic Natural Products (Fortchemie). *Springer*.

CHAPTER FIVE

1. Sanchez, A. Reeser, J. Lau, H. et al., (1973) 'The role of sugars in human neutrophilic phagocytosis' *The American Journal of Clinical Nutrition'*. Vol 26. Issue 11. 1180-1184.

2. Schneider, M. (1995) 'Alcohol and Nutrition'. Based on lectures. M.D. Instructor in Medicine. *University of California*.

3. Greber, G. Leader, L. and et al (1994) 'The Effects of Wheat and other Gluten Grains on the Major Symptoms of Irritable Bowel Syndrome' completed research project supervised by Dr Philip Barlow, Dean of the School of Applied Science and Technology, *University of Humberside*.

4. Hayes, P. Fisher, M. Quigley, E. (2014) 'Irritable Bowel Syndrome: The Role of Food in Pathogenesis and Management'. The Journal of Gastroenterology and Hepatology. NY. Mar. 2014; 10(3): 164-174.

5. Triantafyllidi, A. Xanthos, T. et al., (2015) 'Herbal and Plant Therapy in Patients with Inflammatory Bowel Disease'. Annals of Gastroenterology. 2015 Apr-Jun; 28(2): 210-220.

6. Rao, R. Samak, G. (2011) 'The Role of Glutamine in Protection of Intestinal Epithelial Tight Junctions'. Journal of EpithelioBioPharmacol.2012 Jan; 5 (Supplement 1-M7): 47-54. doi:0.2174/1875044301205010047.

7. Forsyth, P. Bienenstock, J. Kunze, W. (2014) 'Vagal Pathways for Microbiome – Brain – Gut Axis Communication'. Abstract Adv ExpMedBiol 2014; 817:115-33. doi: 10.1007978-1-4939-0897-4-5.

8. Meyer, U. et al., (2014) 'Gut Vagal Efferent Differentially Modulate Innate Anxiety and Learned Fear'. May 21.2014. Journal of Neuroscience 34(21) 7067 -7076. doi: org/10.1523/JNEUROSCI.0252 -14.2014.

9. Konturek, P. et al., (2011) 'Gut Clock: Implication of Circadian Rhythm in the Gastrointestinal Tract'. Review article, Journal of Physiology and Pharmacology 2011.62.2.139-150.

10. Breus, M. (2017) 'Unlocking the Sleep-Gut Connection'. Huffington Post. Healthy Living, new research on sleep and the world of the microbiome. Jan 13, 2017.

11. Ali, T. Choe, J. Awab, A. et al., (2013) 'Sleep, Immunity and Inflammation in Gastrointestinal Disorders'. Journal of World Gastroenterology. 2013 Dec 28; 19(48): 9231-9239. Doi: 10.3748/ wjgv19.i48.9231.

CHAPTER SIX

1. Ritz, E. Hahn, K. et al., (2012) 'Phosphate Additives in Food – a Health Risk'. Deutsches Ärzteblatt International 2012 Jan; 109 (4)

49-55. doi: 10.3238/ärztebl.2012. 0049. NCBI, US National Library of Medicine.

2. Lai, P. Roy, J. (2004) 'Antimicrobial and Chemo-preventive Properties of Herbs and Spices'. Article 2004, *Department of Bioscience, Salem International University* USA. *Current Medicinal Chemistry*, Vol 11, Issue 11. 1451-1460(10). doi: https://doi.org/10.2174/0929867043365107.

3. Cowan, M. (1999) 'Plant Products as Antimicrobial Agents'. *Journal of Clinical Microbiology*. (Reviews) Oct 1999. Vol 12 (4): 564 -582.

4. Pandey, K. Rizvi, S. (2009) 'Plant Polyphenols as dietary Antioxidants in Human Health and Disease'. *Oxidative Medicine and Cellular Longevity*. 2009 Nov-Dec 2(5): 270-278, doi: 10 4161/oxim.2.59498.

5. Willemsen, L. Koetsier, A. Balvers, M et al., (2008) Polyunsaturated Fatty Acids Support Epithelial Barrier Integrity and Reduce IL-4 Mediated Permeability' *Euro J Nutr* 2008; 47(4): 183-191.

6. Calder, P. (2010)' Omega 3 Fatty Acids and Inflammatory Processes' - (online) doi: 10.3390/nu2030355. Cited *PMCID* 3257651.

7. Rapin, J. Wiernsperger, N. (2010) 'Possible Links Between Intestinal Permeability and Food Processing: A Potential Therapeutic Niche for Glutamine'. *San Paolo Clinic*. 2010 Jun; 65(6): 635-643. Doi: 10. 1590/51807-59322010000600012.

8. Garth, L. Nicholson, G. Ash, M. (2014) 'Lipid Replacement Therapy: A Natural Medicine Approach to Replacing Damaged Lipids in Cell Membranes and Organelles and Restoring Function'. *Elsevier, Science Direct*. Biochimica et Biophysica Acta (BBA)-Biomembranes. Vol 1838, Issue 6, June 2014, 1657-1679.

9. Levine, S. (2012) 'Repair the Membrane, Restore the Body'. *Allergy Research Group* Newsletter August 2012.

10. Resnick, C. (2010) 'Nutritional Protocol for the Treatment of Intestinal Permeability Defects and Related Condition'. *Journal of*

Natural Medicine. Mar 2010 Vol 2, Issue 3.

11. Sinn, D. Song, J. Kim, H. et al., (2008) 'Therapeutic Effect of Lactobacillus acidophilus in Patients with Irritable Bowel Disease'. SDC 2012,2013, *Dig Dis Science* 2008 Oct; 53 (10): 2714-8.

12. Williams, A. Simpson, J. Wong, D, et al., (2009) 'Clinical Trial: A Multi Strain Probiotic Preparation Significantly Reduces Symptoms of Irritable Bowel Syndrome'. *Aliment Pharmacology Therapy, Pub Med*, 2009 Jan; 29(1): 97-103.

CHAPTER SEVEN

1. Percival, M. (1997) 'Phytonutrients and Detoxification'. Clinical Nutrition Insights. *The Foundation for the Advancement of Nutritional Education.*

2. Hodges, R. Minich, D. (2015) 'Modulation of Metabolic Detoxification Pathways using Foods and Food-Derived Components: A Scientific Review with Clinical Application'. *Journal of Clinical Nutrition and Metabolism*, Vol 2015, Article ID 76068923.doi. org/10.1155/2015/760689.

3. Allen, J. Montalto M. et al., (2010) 'Detoxification in Naturopathic Medicine: A Survey'. *Journal of Alternative and Complementary Medicine*, Article 2011 Dec; 17(12): 1175-1180, doi: 10.1089/acm.2010.0572.

4. Tisserand, R. (1998) 'Aromatherapy for Everyone', ISBN 0 14 01. 9270 0. *Arkana Penguin Group.*

5. Chaitow, L. (1999) 'Hydrotherapy'. Health Essential Series. *Element Books.*

CHAPTER EIGHT

1. Grandjean, P. (2017)'Human Health Implications of Organic Food and Organic Agriculture' Report for European Parliament. Feb

8, 2017. Co-Authored by Chan, T. School of Public Health. Harvard. *University of Southern Denmark.*

2. Leifert, C. (2015) 'Organic vs Non-Organic Food'. *British Journal of Nutrition.* Study, Oct 2015. Newcastle University.

3. Largest International Study on benefits of Organic Food, based on 200 International Studies. 2016. *British Journal of Nutrition.*

4. Roth-Walter, F. Berin, M. et al., (2008) 'Pasteurisation of Milk Protein Promotes Allergic Sensitisation by Enhancing Uptake Through Peyers Parches'. 2008 *Allergy.* Jul; 63 (7): 882-90, doi:10.11 11/j.1398-9995.2008.01673. x.

5. Bordoni, A. Danesi, F. et al., (2014) 'Dairy Produce and Inflammation: A Review of The Clinical Evidence'. *Journal of Critical Reviews. Food Science and Nutrition.* Vol 57 2017, Issue 12: 2497-2525. Doi.org/10.1080/10408398.2014.967385.

6.Walia, A (2014) 'The Truth About Genetically Modified Food: Know Your Facts'. April 2014. *Scientific American.* Vol 309, Issue 3.

7. Pesticide Action Network UK.' (2013) 'Pesticides on your plate and in your daily bread'. 2013 www.pan-uk.org.

8. Zhou, J. Erdman, J. (2009) 'Phytic Acid in Health and Disease'. *Journal of Critical Reviews in Food Science and Nutrition.* Vol 35, Issue 6: 495-508. doi.org/10.1080/10408399509527712.

9. De Lorgeril, M. Salen, P. (2014) 'Gluten and wheat intolerance today: are modern wheat strains involved?'. *International Journal of Food sciences and Nutrition.* Vol 65, Issue 5: 577-581.

10. De Punder, L. Bruinboom, L. (2013) 'The Dietary Intake of Wheat and Other Cereal Grains and their Role in Inflammation'. Article cited in *US National Library of Medicine.* 2013 Mar 12, doi: 10.3390/nu5030771.

11. Uhde, M. Ajamian, M. et al., (2016) 'Intestinal Cell Damage and Systemic Immune Activation in Individuals Reporting Sensitivity to Wheat in the Absence of Coeliac Disease'. Original article Gut online 10.1136/gutjnl2016-311964, *group.bmj.com* July 2016.

12. Kucek, L. Veenstra. et al., (2015) 'A Grounded Guide to Gluten: How Modern Genotypes and Processing Impact Wheat Sensitivity'. *Wiley online library*. Feb 2015, doi:10.1111/14541 -4337.12129, Vol 14, Issue TOC, May 2015: 285-302.

CHAPTER NINE

1. Vance, E. (2016) 'Mind Over Matter' Dec 2016: 30-55. *National Geographic Magazine*.

Resources

LIST OF LABORATORIES:

Biolab Medical Unit
The Stone House
9 Weymouth Street
Marylebone, London WIW 6DB, UK
Tel: (+44) 020 7636 5959/5905
Email: reception@biolab.co.uk
Offer a range of gastrointestinal and nutritional testing procedures

Genova Diagnostics UK
46-50 Coombe Road
New Malden, Surrey KT3 4QF, UK
Tel: (+44) 20 8336 7750
Email: kitorders@gdx.net
Offer a range of gastrointestinal and nutritional profiles

Regenerus Laboratories (Cyrex Tests)
Aero 14 Kings Mill Lane
Redhill, Surrey RH1 5JH, UK
Tel: (+44) 203 7500870
Email: info@regeneruslabs.com
Offers a range of current specialised food intolerance and cross reactivity tests

Invivo Clinical Laboratory Diagnostics and Nutraceuticals
Unit 1, The New Warehouse
Libby's Drive 3
Stroud, Gloucestershire GL5 IRN, UK
Tel: (+44) 0 333241 2997
Practitioner only email support@invivoclinical.co.uk
Offers Advanced Intestinal Barrier Assessment

Doctor's Data Inc
3755 Illinois Avenue
St Charles IL 60174-2420, USA
UK contact 0871 218 0052
Email: info@doctorsdata.com
Offers a range of intestinal profiles in Clinical Microbiology

Contacts

The Institute for Optimum Nutrition
Ambassador House
Paradise Road, Richmond
London TW9 1SQ, UK
Tel: (+44) 0208 614 7800
Email: info@ion.ac.uk, website www.ion.ac.uk
Training courses
Onsite Clinic offering Consultations and Laboratory testing.
Practitioner register.

CNELM -The Centre for Nutrition Education
and Lifestyle Management
Chapel Garden, 14 Rectory Road
Wokingham, Berks RG40 1DH, UK
Tel: (+44) 0118 979 8686
Email: info@cnelm.co.uk
Graduate and Post graduate training courses. Practitioner list.

The Institute for Functional Medicine
505 S 336th Street Suite 600
Federal Way. WA. 98003, USA
Tel: 1. 800.228. 0622
Functional Medicine Courses and Practitioner list.
UK Contact: Clinical Education www.clinicaleducation.org IFM
Collaboration

The Heidelberg Test for stomach acid (pH Test)
Information: jonbarron.org/article/testyourstomachacid
The Baseline of Health Foundation
Advice: contact GP for resource information

Mineral Check
Bull Cottage
Lenham Heath Road
Maidstone, **Kent** ME17 2BP, UK
Tel: (+44) 01622 850 500
Email: mineralcheck@mineralcheck.com
Hair Mineral Analysis

BANT
The British Association for Applied Nutrition and Nutritional Therapy
The Professional Body for Nutritional Therapists
27 Old Gloucester Street
London WC1N 3XX, UK
Tel: 0870 606 1284
Practitioner register
Email: the administrator@bant.org.uk

NUTRITIONAL SUPPLEMENTS:

THE NATURAL DISPENSARY
Libby's Drive
Slad Road
Stroud, **Gloucestershire** GL5 1RN, UK
Tel: (+44) 01453 75 77 92
Email: enquiries@naturaldispensary.co.uk

BIONUTRI
1 Beech Road
Bourneville
Birmingham B30 9LL, UK
Tel: (+44) 0121 628 1901
Email: info@bionutri.co.uk

NUTRI-LINK
Nutrition House, 24 Milber Lane Trading Estate
Newton Abbot
Devon TQ 12 4SG, UK
Tel: (+44) 0333 241 4289
www.nutri-link.co.uk
The Gastro Test.
Tel: 08458 949767

There are many excellent box schemes that deliver fresh organic produce direct from the farm to your home: Riverhead Farm, Abel & Cole, Eversfield, Ocado, Farmaround. As many are franchised, it is best to look locally for your contact number.

Naturally leavened organic healthy bread is available. https://theartisanbakery.com operate a home delivery scheme and have some interesting gluten-free grain breads from rice, pea, buckwheat, quinoa, linseed combinations; it is well worth looking at their site. Flour and Spoon also deal with naturally leavened bread.

Farmers Markets, though not all affording the Soil Association Accreditation, can supply organic produce, local cheeses, yoghurts and a range of unprocessed foods.

ACKNOWLEDGEMENTS

Credit is due to many renowned writers and researchers in the field of Nutritional and Functional Medicine who have influenced my thinking and provided significant inspiration in my working life: Dr Jeffrey Bland, Dr Linus Pauling, Dr Carl Pfeiffer, Assistant Professor Melvyn Werbach, M.D. Assistant Clinical Professor, Joseph Pizzorno, N.D. Michael Murray, N.D. Weston A. Price, D.D.S. and Alfred Vogel, Swiss Naturopath.

I thank the many patients with often challenging difficult medical histories, who through compliance and determination enhanced my knowledge and understanding.

Grateful thanks go to my sons Damon and Marcus and supportive family for comments, thoughts and being there for me; to my caring husband for giving me unlimited space to write in peace and quiet and special thanks to my daughter Nicole and son-in-law Marc for endless patience, good advice and design work.

I am indebted to my brother Terry Robinson, Technical Author for providing images, valuable technical advice and for proof reading.

Thank also to my friend and colleague Fleur Brown from The Institute For Optimum Nutrition study days for boosting morale with constructive chats.

Bibliography

FURTHER READING:

Richard A. Passwater, Elmer M. Cranton, *Trace Elements, Hair Mineral Analysis and Nutrition:* Keats Publishing USA 1983. ISBN 0-87983-265-7

Carl C. Pfeiffer, *Mental and Elemental Nutrients*: Keats Publishing, USA 1975. ISBN 0-97983-114-6

Maria C. Linder, *Nutritional Biochemistry and Metabolism*: Appleton & Lange USA, 1991. ISBN 0-8385-7084-4

Elizabeth Lipski, *Digestive Wellness*: Keats Publishing USA 2000. ISBN second edition 0-87983-984-8

Patrick Holford, *The Optimum Nutrition Bible*: Piatkus Reprint, London, 2009. ISBN 978-0-7499-2552-9

Paul Clayton, *Health Defence*, UK: Accelerated Learning Systems Ltd, UK, 2001. ISBN 0-905553 63 2

D. Lindsey Berkson, *Healthy Digestion the Natural Way*: John Wiley & Sons Inc, USA, 2000. ISBN 0-471-34962-3

Thomas Bartram, *The Encyclopaedia of Herbal Medicine*: Grace Publishers UK, 1995. ISBN 0-9515984-1-4

Alfred Vogel, *The Nature Doctor*, Switzerland: Verlag A Vogel(AR), reprinted 2007. ISBN 978 1851582747

William L. Wolcott, *The Metabolic Typing Diet*: Doubleday, USA a division of Random House, 2000. ISBN 0-385-49691-5

Readers Digest, *Foods That Harm, Foods that Heal*, UK: The Readers Digest Association Limited, 2002. ISBN 0 276 42673 8

Bill Gottlieb, *Alternative Cures:* Rodale Inc. USA. ISBN 1-57954-058-9. 2000

Elson M. Haas, *Staying Healthy with Nutrition, The Complete Guide to Diet and Nutritional Medicine:* CelestiaL Arts Publishing. Berkeley, California USA. ISBN 0-89087- 481-6. 1992.

Selene Yeager and the Editors of Prevention Health Books, *New Foods for Healing*: Rodale Press Inc. Pennsylvania. USA 1998. ISBN 0-87596-413-3

Jill Scott, *Healing Food*: Hermes House, Anness Publishing Limited. London. 2000, 2004. CIP Catalogue at British Library.

Leon Chaitow, *Natural Alternatives to Antibiotic*: Thorsons, an imprint of Harper Collins Publishers. London, 1998. ISBN 0 00 712247 0

Phyllis A. Balch, *Prescription for Nutritional Healing*: Avery, a member of Penguin Putnam Inc. New York. USA 2000. ISBN 1-58333-077-1

Michael Murray and Joseph Pizzorno, *Encyclopaedia of Natural Medicine*: Three Rivers Press. New York. USA. 1997. ISBN 0-7615-1157-1

Melvyn R. Werbach, *Nutritional Influences on Illness*: Keats publishing Inc. Connecticut. 1987. ISBN 0-87983-500-1

Jean Carper, *Food Your Miracle Medicine*: Simon & Schuster of Australia Pty Ltd. 1994. ISBN 0-671-71336-1

Dicken Weatherby and Scott Ferguson, *Blood Chemistry and CBC Analysis – Clinical Laboratory Testing from a Functional Perspective*: Vis Medicatrix Press. USA. 2002. ISBN 0-9726469-0-6

M. F. Laker, *Clinical Biochemistry*: W. B. Saunders Company Limited. London. 1996. ISBN 0-7020-1690-X

Laz Bannock, *Clinical Human Nutrition*: Human Nutrition.com. 2002. ISBN o-9542017-0-1

Ralph Golan, *Optimal Wellness*: Ballantine Books, New York. 1995. ISBN 0-345-35874-09

Gayla J. Kirschmann and John D. Kirschmann, *Nutrition Almanac:* McGraw-Hill. New York. 1973, reprinted in PP 1996. ISBN 0-07-034922-3

Geoffrey Cannon, *The Politics of Food*: Century. London. 1987. ISBN 0-7126-1210-6

Weston A. Price, *Nutrition and Physical Degeneration*: Keats Publishing USA. Reprinted 1997. ISBN 0-87983-816-7

Drs Stephan Davies and Alan Stewart, *Nutritional Medicine*: Pan Books, London. 1987. ISBN 0 350 28833 4

Dr Bernard Jenson, *Foods that Heal*: Avery Publishing Group. New York. 1993. ISBN 0-89529-563-6

James Braly M.D. *Food Allergy and Nutrition Revolution*: Keats Publishing USA. 1992. ISBN 0-87983-590-7

Lynne McTaggart, *What Doctors Don't Tell You*: Thorsons. London. 1996. ISBN 0 7225 3024 2

Martin J. Walker, *Dirty Medicine*: Slingshot Publications. London. 1993. ISBN 0 9519646 0 7

Index

163, 164, 167, 168, 169, 171,
182, 183, 188, 189, 196, 198,
200, 201, 210, 211, 214, 217,
218, 225, 231, 233, 235, 236,
237, 238, 253

protein whey 183

psyllium fibre formula 142

pyloric sphincter 38

Pyroluria (urine) 70

pyrroles 70

Q

quick and easy biscuits 243

quick and easy cakes 242

quick and easy treats 243

quinoa 89, 102, 103, 128, 218,
239, 259

R

recommended dietary
allowances (RDA) 26

recommended FM tests 134,
139, 143, 147, 150, 153, 155

recommended nutritional
supplements 134

red blood cells 21, 200

red wine 15

reflux esophagitis 45, 248

regression whilst progressing
222

regular eating pattern 48

root vegetables 68, 87, 113, 124,
136, 141, 144, 150, 152, 155,

158, 159, 161, 163, 183

Roundup (herbicide) 211, 212

rye 83, 84, 89, 103, 107, 148,
179, 216, 218, 242

S

salivary amylase 39, 46

saliva test 66

saunas 204, 205

secretin 47

secretory immunoglobulin A (s
IgA) 66

secretory immunoglobulin A (s
IgA) (saliva test) 66

selenium 16, 18, 24, 25, 42, 190,
196, 201

self-heal 22

self-help 14, 116, 127, 130, 157,
159, 161, 163, 164, 165, 167,
169, 171, 224, 244

self-help treatment plans 116,
127

serum blood test 65, 67

SIBO breath test (small
intestinal bacterial
overgrowth) 71

signs of bacterial infection 80

signs of poor liver function 199

skin 4, 5, 21, 23, 24, 25, 27, 28,
43, 44, 47, 68, 70, 78, 80, 81,
82, 102, 118, 131, 132, 146,
148, 151, 170, 184, 186, 199,
200, 204, 205, 208, 213, 233

204

vitamin A 25, 27, 124, 137, 145, 151, 154, 155, 156, 183, 196, 205, 206, 218

vitamin B 25, 31

vitamin B complex 25

vitamin C 8, 15, 16, 21, 23, 24, 25, 26, 27, 31, 34, 51, 52, 53, 54, 69, 70, 96, 99, 109, 124, 134, 148, 151, 154, 156, 159, 160, 165, 167, 168, 170, 187, 196, 200, 201, 236

vitamin D 25, 27, 51, 162, 169, 170, 171, 205

vitamin E 25, 27, 124, 184, 196, 217

vitamin K 25, 79, 124, 183, 191

vitamin profile (blood serum test) 72

vitamins and minerals 72, 96, 168, 196, 206, 217, 218

W

walnuts 95, 163, 182, 186, 198, 235, 239, 242

water 7, 18, 21, 33, 35, 40, 44, 49, 50, 52, 54, 75, 82, 83, 84, 87, 90, 94, 97, 100, 108, 109, 112, 114, 121, 125, 126, 127, 130, 140, 148, 150, 159, 160, 164, 167, 169, 176, 179, 192, 194, 195, 196, 198, 200, 204, 214, 222, 230, 232, 233, 240, 241, 242

wheat 68, 69, 72, 74, 84, 87, 92, 93, 94, 95, 101, 103, 108, 110, 112, 118, 120, 121, 127, 129, 131, 134, 147, 148, 150, 160, 175, 177, 179, 214, 215, 216, 217, 218, 235, 238, 239, 240, 249, 253, 254

white blood cells 21, 67, 76, 89, 119, 236

wholegrain rice 114, 128, 157, 184, 238, 239

wholegrains 60, 61, 84, 87, 95, 118, 120, 159, 161, 162, 166, 167, 169, 171, 175, 194, 213, 214, 231, 237

Y

yeast 11, 15, 65, 66, 67, 68, 76, 80, 81, 83, 84, 95, 101, 112, 113, 146, 147, 148, 160, 161, 240, 241

yeast culture 67, 147

yeast culture (stool test) 67, 147

yeast infestation 80

Z

zinc 8, 15, 16, 17, 18, 23, 28, 31, 42, 53, 69, 70, 73, 93, 95, 96, 104, 106, 109, 114, 118, 119, 120, 127, 129, 134, 137, 145, 151, 154, 156, 166, 167, 168, 170, 187, 188, 190, 196, 213, 218

zinc methionine 69

Printed in Great Britain
by Amazon